Liberation

Secrets of the Soul

Lina Girgis

Short Stories

Title: Liberation: Secrets of the Soul, Short Stories
Author: Lina Girgis

First edition

5.25" x 8"

214 pages
Approx. 59,000 words

Bookman 10/14
Papyrus 20
Optima 8

Cover painting: Lina Girgis

Editing and design
Danielle Aubrey
Peter Geldart

Petra Books
petrabooks.ca

I hope you enjoy reading my book and consider writing a review on Amazon.

Lina

Dedication

To my mother, my creator
To my father, my comforter
To my sister, my soulmate
To my son, my strength
To my daughter, my inspiration

Destiny lets your soul be shattered,
so the scattered pieces eventually reunite
to form a mosaic of your beautiful portrait
and orchestrate your unique life symphony.
Only at the climax will you figure out
your own story.

— Lina Girgis

Table of Contents

A Glimpse Inward

All her life she had been looking for a soulmate who could sense her unspoken thoughts and embrace her unexpressed feelings — rather than merely a heart to love her, or an eye to covet her, let alone a body to use hers. She contemplated this old yearning — hidden in her head, refusing to lose hope, yet clinging to very little of it — while making coffee in the early morning.

This Saturday was special. She was going to meet her old friend who was in Ottawa on a business trip for a couple of days. Alena could not believe her eyes when she had read Nour's letter two days earlier; they had not written to each other for about fifteen years. Thankfully, Nour had mailed it early, as it took a month for the letter to arrive at Alena's new address. Otherwise, she would have missed Nour's visit altogether. It was a surprise that shook the comfortable routine of Alena's life. She was eager to see Nour and listen to her news. After all these years, Nour would surely have plenty of amusing stories to tell. For Alena, however, it would be awkward to find something to talk about. Where would she even start?

She sat at the round kitchen table, turned the radio on — her only connection with the outer world — and breathed the fresh earthy scent of petrichor. Alena listened attentively to the news, and then changed from the local to the international station. It was time for the musical Turkish program. Although she did not understand the lyrics, she still enjoyed the tunes. The songs reminded her of life itself — a beautiful melody with words written in a language she did not fully comprehend.

Still wet from her morning shower, her wavy hair was free to dry by nature's breath. The herbal scent of shampoo, blending with the aroma of hot coffee, filled the room. The window curtain and tablecloth, patterned with fruits and vegetables on an amber background, swayed in the breeze to the musical wind chimes. The window overlooked a quiet path, lined with tall white spruce trees, which lead to a gazebo in the middle of a public garden.

She finished coffee and tended to her best friend — the indoor jasmine tree that stood in the corner of her kitchen. She watered the soothing plant gently, talking to the leaves to say good morning. The fragrance of jasmine dreamily carried her back home; there, in the backyard of the five-storey apartment building where she grew up, was a much bigger jasmine tree.

Satisfied with how she looked in the mirror, she placed a pink scarf which matched her lipstick around her shoulders. Grabbing the car keys, she headed for down-town. They were meeting for breakfast at the Baker Street Café which was walking distance from the Ottawa River. She spent the half-hour drive thinking about stories from her past, and the many people she had known in Egypt before she had left forever. She had so many questions for Nour about her and their friends, whom she had not seen or heard from for decades.

She had been thinking about Nour's visit since the previous night, bringing back memories — memories as old as her grandmother. Doris and her fiancé had moved from Athens to Alexandria after World War I — a war that had destroyed a great deal of Europe's beauty and security. When both she and the century were in their early twenties, Doris, along with many Europeans, came to Egypt to start a new life and to seek refuge in this safe, elegant, and developed country. Back then.

Doris, her paternal grandmother, was the only reason Alena could still remember a few Greek words — she always spoke to her in Greek. However Leila, Alena's mother, born to an Egyptian mother and a Greek father, did not speak one word of Greek. Neither Leila nor Panos, Alena's father, had ever seen Greece; neither of their families could afford the flight tickets at the time. World War II erupted while they were teenagers and continued until they were in their early twenties. They were shielded in Egypt, even though Alexandria was not so far from the battlefields. After all, they were both born and raised in Alexandria, and though Leila's blood was half Egyptian, her soul was entirely so.

Alena recalled Sunday mornings, when her grandmother took her and her sister to the Greek Orthodox Cathedral in Alexandria. After nearly every mass, they would walk by the ancient Mediterranean Sea. She loved listening to the waves which mingled with her grandmother's soft voice as she told tales of her beloved country on the opposite shore.

Alena experienced the strongest Greek influence through her paternal grandparents, yet she also felt a close connection with her Egyptian culture. Her exposure to the Greek culture ended with her grandmother's death when she was in high school, while her Egyptian culture expanded from her birth and during her youth, until she decided to come to Canada. She grew up the same way as the other Egyptian children, among whom she barely felt different. Later, during her years at university and at work, she did not experience the persecution, unlike many Christians in

Egypt. Most of her close friends were Muslim, one of whom was Nour.

Soaked in her sweet and sour memories, Alena found herself downtown Ottawa, only two blocks away from the coffee shop. She parked her small car and walked for five minutes. She loved to walk under the gentle autumn sun as she gazed at the amazing colours of the leaves. She contemplated the paradoxical beauty of the trees and their leaves, growing old and dying around her.

Arriving early, she entered the small bistro and asked for a table for two. Leaving her purse on the opposite seat, she sat down and began to look around and observe people — her favoured hobby of all time. There was a young woman sitting by herself, worried and confused, looking at her watch every second, until her long-awaited knight showed up, apologising many times for being late and providing his excuses. They fell into a hot, romantic dialogue full of emotions, dreams, and promises.

Alena was taken to their little world, as they were building together their charming sand castle on the non-existing beach of their unknown future. *It's just the beginning; any love story starts with the same words and repeated promises — every time, everywhere,* she thought. *I wonder how it's going to end though.*

While Alena was lost in thought, Nour arrived looking for her, and when she saw her, she walked toward the table and burst into her well-known, loud laughter.

"Seriously, Alena, you still drown absentmindedly in your deep thoughts, like you always did," Nour teased her.

Her laughter distracted Alena's contemplation, and she jumped from her seat. They held each other tight for as long as the many years that separated them, until their eyes sparkled with tears. They stared at each other for a few seconds, until they both uttered at the very same moment, "You haven't changed a bit."

Nour sat down on the opposite chair. As always, Nour took the initiative and said, "Alena, I haven't realised how much I missed you until now. You have kids. Right?"

"Yes, I have Youssef and Rashi. They both go to McGill University in Montreal."

"And how is Magued?"

Alena stayed silent for a few seconds, and then answered, "I'm sure he's doing very well." She fiddled with one of her square sky-blue topaz earrings that matched the tint of her eye shadow.

"What do you mean?" Nour asked.

"Magued and I got divorced a few years ago." Alena smoothed her brown outfit.

"What? I can't believe it. After your famous fairy-tale love story?" Nour questioned.

"Oh yes, believe it. There's nothing in this world too hard to believe," replied Alena, having trouble maintaining eye contact.

"But why?" asked wide-eyed Nour.

"The minutiae of daily life." Alena took the scarf off from around her neck and hung it on the back of the chair.

"The minutiae of daily life!" Nour echoed Alena in confused shock; she expected to hear that there had been another woman, or a long story with as much suspense as she saw in movies or read in books. She could hardly believe that reality was much simpler than she could imagine. Wondering what Alena meant by that, Nour asked, "What do you mean?"

"I couldn't live with him in the same house or share the same kind of life any longer. He had his own way of living that made him feel comfortable, and so did I. The problem was that the two ways were different. And it's not fair to force the lifestyle you choose on someone else to the point that it turns their life into hell."

"Did he leave you so easily?" Nour asked.

"Of course not. No man leaves a woman just like that, even if he doesn't want her. A man usually considers his woman as one of his possessions," said Alena in a cracked tone, her eyes avoiding and trying to escape the subject.

Alena and Magued had met when she started her first job. Marrying an Egyptian was no issue, because she always considered herself as one. Then one year after their marriage, they both felt that Egypt was not the place they wanted to raise their children. Egypt was no longer the beautiful, safe country to which her grandparents had fled fifty years earlier.

In the 1970s Egypt became financially challenging and economically discouraging for the new generations. The Islamic ideologists' influence, creeping from the newly-rich neighbouring country that dominated the Arabian Peninsula, gradually conquered the Egyptian soil. And the Islamic extremists' views found their secret ways to penetrate the Egyptian soul.

Alena and Magued felt like strangers in their own land. She thought of moving to Greece, but Magued had a broader vision, which she happened to like. Finally, they ended up in peaceful Canada, where they had both of their children, and where Alena lived, satisfied until that day.

Surely, there was so much to say about the reasons for their divorce, but Alena preferred to keep it all to herself, especially since those stories were already fading away in her memory. She was not interested in bringing them back to life. In an attempt to broach a new subject, Alena looked at Nour and asked, "Tell me now, do you have children?" Alena's brown eyes smiled, curled thick eyelashes framed them.

"I never got married in the first place," Nour answered.

"How come? You mentioned in your last letter that you were engaged." Alena's forehead puckered.

"Yes, I was. We broke up, and since then, I haven't met my one-and-only yet. If I had been married, I wouldn't have reached my present position at work. My life revolves around work. I am the Regional Director of Marketing and Public Relations at one of the largest investment corporations in the Middle East," said Nour, as her fingers formed a steeple.

"You're right. When a woman gets married and has children, she spends all her time caring for her family and home," said Alena, twisting her ring. "Still, some women can do both at the same time. I don't know how, though."

"I know how. They get all the support and help from their husbands."

"I can only focus on one thing. That's why I spent all my life taking care of my children. Although my time wasn't wasted, sadly this is exactly how I feel now," confessed Alena, looking down at the table. "I work with the city; it's a decent job, for which I'm thankful."

"You know something," Nour said, "I don't really care for getting married or being in a relationship anymore; what I truly miss is not having my own son or daughter."

"Children are a gift from Heaven, but once they grow up and become independent, it's over. What I mean is, having children won't make a big difference in the end. Look at me! I have a girl and a boy, but I also live alone. I

soon realised that I am the best company for myself."
Alena pressed her hands to her cheeks.

"I can't say that I'm lonely. As you know, I can't live
without people. Half of my life is for work, and the other
half is with family and friends," said Nour, lifting her
head, "yet having my own children would be something
else. How about you? Do you have friends here in Canada?"

"For sure, I know many people in Ottawa, but at the
end of the day, everyone is busy with their own lives."

They paused to skim through the menu quietly until
both were ready to order the food. And soon their
breakfast was served on the table. For a little while,
silence prevailed; each of them examined the other
secretly. Alena scanned Nour's face; she noticed that her
hair was bleached; she had never seen her blonde before.
Did she bleach it just for a change or to cover the grey hair?
she silently wondered. Alena also observed that Nour's
face was relaxed, with close to no wrinkles, unlike hers.
*Maybe because she never got pregnant or stayed up long
sleepless nights*, pondered Alena.

Similarly, Nour inspected Alena in silence, looking at
her from the corners of her eyes as she ate. Alena looked
as she always had: simple, elegant, and pretty. Nour
noticed that Alena's hair was not dyed. Alena had lived all
her life with her natural hair colour, and she did not mind
the appearance of some grey. Her hair was almost-black
dark brown in the indoor light, but the sun's rays added a
burgundy tone to it. It was the colour of eggplant, and it
deliciously enhanced her olive skin.

Nour saw that Alena's eyes still had the same continuous
bewilderment and mysterious embarrassment. And while
Nour was a good speaker — grabbing people's attention by
her talk and laughter — she was now wondering how to

resume the conversation; she was looking for the right question to ask or subject to open. Alena, who rarely spoke, preferred to rather listen and contemplate profoundly.

"Is there a man in your life?" asked a curious Nour.

"No, there isn't. They're all friends," Alena admitted.

"Why just friends?"

"Less complicated that way. How about you?" Alena asked.

"I've met many men in my life, but the story ends there every time. And the older I get, the harder it is. Now, I have my position at work, my own house and a lifestyle that I've chosen for myself. It's hard to find a suitable man who deserves that I sacrifice any of that. So, for me, it's the same; they're all just friends." Nour shrugged.

"I totally understand because I have very similar circumstances. And sometimes being alone can be a blessing. Tell me, then, have you ever thought of leaving Egypt and moving elsewhere?"

"I could never leave Egypt." Nour's lips stretched in a confident smile. "What are you talking about? Why would I? I'd be like a fish out of water. In my eyes, Egypt is the most beautiful country in the world." She sipped some of her apple juice.

"I'm surprised. Egypt was a prison for me: an intellectual, emotional, and social prison," Alena recalled slowly as she sliced up the crepes.

"I feel like you're talking about another Egypt," Nour reflected, adding some pepper to her omelette. "But are you happy here? I mean, you'll never be Canadian, after all. You'll always be looked upon as an immigrant."

"Well, I didn't choose how I look, where I was born or grew up, or who my parents were. What I chose was to come to Canada to start a new life," Alena answered Nour, looking her in the eyes. "What makes me Canadian is not my skin colour or English accent, but whether or not I share and respect Canadian values. My kids are Canadian. Canada is my home now."

Alena was indifferent to being Egyptian — neither ashamed nor proud, and she considered it a fact of life that she had never been given the opportunity to choose her birthplace. What she sensed with certainty was that she did not fit in Egyptian society.

Nothing in the world frustrated her more than the unfair, huge social gap dividing the country into a remarkably rich minority, an extremely poor majority, and a vanishing middle class. Good education and health care were provided only to those who could afford to pay thousands of Pounds, leaving the vast majority of people with no choice but to attend corrupt public schools and to seek treatment at neglected public hospitals.

Growing levels of poverty and illiteracy worsened the backward mentality and social traditions which belittled women in the Middle Eastern cultures. Corruption spread like cancer in the country on all levels and in every domain. The stubborn mind-set of many could not accept different beliefs and ruined even the most intimate relationships among friends and neighbours.

Alena had no desire to go back, not even for a visit. None of her family remained — her parents had passed away, and Liliana, her only sister, had decided to move with her own small family to Toronto two years later. Alena did not have family in Greece either.

When Alena first moved to Ottawa, she had found it easy to adjust to the Canadian traditions. The Canadian culture appealed to her, language being no barrier. Yet even now she did not completely mingle in the Canadian world. At times, she still felt like an outsider.

Never in her entire life did she find a tribe she wished to be part of or a land to belong to; there was always something missing. She was too Egyptian and Middle-Eastern to be Greek, too modern and practical to be Egyptian, and too sophisticated and Mediterranean to be Canadian. Sometimes it felt so confusing that she surely must have been born on the wrong planet or perhaps in a mistaken century.

Time flew, and before they knew it, lunch was over. Nour, looking at her watch, realised it was time to go; she had to be at the airport in two hours to catch her flight back to Cairo. Her business trip was over, and it had ended with the sweetest opportunity to see Alena and spend some precious moments with her. They hugged and promised they would always stay in touch until another occasion would unite them once more. Each one went her way.

Alena drove back home in her car. Turning on the radio, she was disturbed that they were still discussing the causes of a recent airline crash. Most of the news was about the conflict in the Middle East. Then, another news item discussed the Y2K crisis that would face the world by the beginning of the year 2000. *How depressing this world is becoming* she thought, turning off the radio with a trembling hand. She wondered whether the new millennium would bring any joy to this miserable world, or would it only add more hatred, insecurity, and distrust.

She considered Nour's visit, which had shaken the solid ground of her boring life like a major earthquake. She felt lost. She had a longing to go home; she just did not know where home was. Perhaps this encounter with

Nour after all these years had awoken emotions and thoughts inside her that had long been submerged, bringing back memories she had tried to avoid. She rather felt herself in the spotlight as she began to rethink her entire life. It made her think about 'Alena'. *Is it too late for me?* she asked herself.

She questioned if she honestly enjoyed her aloneness as she isolated herself from the world, wasting her days. She wondered if she was truly satisfied with her life, or did she passively accept it. She could not believe how fast the years had slipped through her fingers when she tried to remember one thing she did to prove she could succeed in something. The emptiness of her life over the last few years had gradually formed a depressing enclosure of which she was hardly aware. And without noticing, she had given in to the day-to-day stillness of her lifeless routine.

The phone was ringing as she opened the door of her apartment and she ran to answer.

"Hi, Alena. Where have you been all day? I called you six times," Liliana said on the other end.

"Hi Lili. I had an interesting, long visit with Nour, my friend from Alexandria."

"I barely remember her, but that's so cool."

"Yeah, it was nice," said Alena as she laid her purse on the coffee table. "She has a prestigious position with a big corporation. She never got married, though. I was surprised."

"Interesting!"

"But she's happy. She has a wonderful career." Alena sank into the armchair.

"How are your other two friends?" Liliana asked.

"Hoda is an English Literature Professor at the University of Alexandria. And Noha moved to England with her husband. She works as a translator," said Alena, her attention captured by the pattern of the rug under her feet.

"Do you have plans for Thanksgiving? Are the kids coming to see you?" Liliana asked.

"No. They're too busy," Alena answered in a flat tone.

"Are you alright?" Liliana wondered.

"It sounds like I'm the only one of them who didn't really accomplish anything," Alena said, playing with her hair.

"You've raised two wonderful people."

"What have I done for myself, though? Nothing! I used my children as an excuse. What did I do with my life? Where did the time go? I've wasted all my life waiting for the right moment to start doing something for myself. And this moment never came."

"You worked. You have a good job."

"But I failed to build a career. I could've done my graduate studies, but I chose not to. My life has been purposeless. I failed my marriage. I'm not even sure I was a good mother."

"Don't be too hard on yourself, Alena. You're a great mother and your children love you. You're not the only woman who got divorced. And it was your wish anyway."

"I never knew what I wanted. Even now, I don't know what I want. My life is tasteless. I need to have a goal. A dream. Something to live for." She rose and walked around as she talked.

"You're smart. You always got the best grades in class. Remember?"

"What have I done with my good grades? Nothing."

"You're talented, Alena. Remember when you decided to paint again?"

"Haven't even started."

"Ask yourself why. Promise yourself this time to start something and finish it."

"I know for sure I'm not stupid. I know I'm not lazy. But I also know that my dilemma is that I don't know what I want. I never cared for academia. Having a career was not my ultimate ambition. A job for me is just something to pay my bills and keep me busy."

"Be thankful then," Liliana said.

"I am thankful, but I'm not fulfilled. There's something missing. I think I can do more. I feel like a part of me is waiting to be discovered. I've wasted my life. There's no one to blame but myself." Alena collapsed into the armchair once more.

"You did the best you could. Stop blaming yourself for everything," said Liliana.

"I feel sorry for myself." Alena wrapped a curl around her finger.

"You need to find a man, Alena," Liliana suggested.

"I need to find myself first," Alena sighed.

Alena ended her phone call, turned on the radio, and started wandering around the apartment. She stopped in front of every picture on the walls. She went through both bedrooms as if she was looking for something. She opened her closet, looked through her clothes and then closed it again. She went to the kitchen and drank a glass of water.

She glanced at the dying sunflowers in the big clay pot on the balcony, drying up under the sun. She stood for a minute, contemplating behind closed glass balcony doors. As she walked by the bathroom, she noticed her figure in the mirror. She stopped, walked closer, and stared at her face and body for a long time. The wrinkles seemed deeper, the grey hair had increased, and her body was heavier than she had last noticed.

She found herself in front of the storage room. It was cluttered with plastic bags of shoes and clothes she had been meaning to donate, and a box of books she still wished to read. Another box was on the shelf, full of video and cassette tapes. Some pictures were stacked behind the boxes against the wall that she had intended to hang but never had. She found the acrylic paint containers, the canvas frames, and the easel she had bought months earlier in the far-left corner. She took the painting materials out and placed them on the dining table.

Already feeling hungry, Alena went to the kitchen, drank water again, and prepared a simple meal for her dinner. In the plate, the avocado, chickpeas, and beets looked like one of the colourful paintings she had painted in the past. The dish smelled like a warm garden. After her small meal, she made her daily hot drink of ginger and cinnamon, turned off the radio, and went to the living room.

The hot, spicy drink brought her blood back to life. She turned on her cassette player to listen to a collection of songs from the sixties. She delighted in the old songs as she admired the tableaux on the walls. Paintings and melodies were the two wings which flew Alena to her firmament of comfort. And the higher she went, the smaller the world appeared in her eyes.

The sage walls of her small apartment were covered with pictures and paintings of all sizes and types: family photos, panoramic sceneries, and vivid paintings by local artists, whom she was always keen on supporting. In her bedroom, a big picture of Queen Cleopatra hung above her bed. On the nightstand lay the book <u>Hypatia of Alexandria</u> next to an elegant, antique lamp.

Trying to warm herself on that cold night, she held the hot cup between her hands and stood in front of the fireplace and her bookshelves, gazing at all the books she had read, trying to remember what each of them was about. There was the Greek mythology collection on the top shelf, next to the Bible, and the <u>Egyptian Book of the Dead</u>. The scent of history revived her soul.

On the second shelf were English literature books from her undergraduate university degree and others: novels, plays, and anthologies. When she saw <u>Mrs. Dalloway</u> by Virginia Woolf, she felt like reading it again. The third shelf had Egyptian and Canadian novels, short story collections, and a few books of poetry. She grabbed <u>Woman at Point Zero</u> by Nawal El Saadawi; she smiled and leafed through some pages and put it back. Next to it stood <u>The Handmaid's Tale</u> by Margaret Atwood.

Getting tired of standing, she went to her desk, sat down, opened the top drawer, and took out her thick notebook in which she wrote every night before going to bed. That night, she chose to read rather than write. She flipped the pages and read lines here and there: some written years earlier, and some, only a few days back. A few forgotten lines made her stop and read them out loud.

The strong woman always looks for a stronger man; the intelligent woman does not mind if her man is more intelligent; the brave woman is pleased to find a man, braver than she is. Is this how things normally are? Is it really an instinct in every woman, as women always convince themselves? Or are they accumulations in the subconscious of humanity, piled up for centuries because of the patriarchal world, which indirectly tells women they are inferior? Where did the goddesses of the ancient civilisations go? Why has the female half of the universe been hidden all these centuries?

Alena glanced at the framed photo of her grandmother and grinned. It was Doris who had named her 'Alena' and always reminded her that her name had a purposeful meaning: protector of humanity, which, to Alena, had not made much sense. *How could anybody protect humanity anyway, and protect it from what or whom* she had wondered. Later, she had learned that her name also meant 'light', which made her wonder more and ask herself if it was light that could protect humanity. "Is it the light of knowledge? Or the light of faith?" she asked. *Or perhaps both* she thought.

Alena took the last sip of her bittersweet drink, closed the notebook, and laid it gently on the desk. She reclined in the chair, contemplating why she could not write for others to share with them her reflections. Staring at her painting materials, she spent a long time conversing internally with herself, diving into her deep soul. She asked questions and searched for answers, striving to pinpoint what type of writing would best fulfil her potential.

And that night, she made the decision which started a new chapter of her life. She would write short stories. *They are condensed, precise, powerful, and quick to read, coping with the fast pace of today's world* she concluded. Literary fiction would allow room for her artistic creativity. Writing a short story would be like painting a scene — a brief period of time, photographed in the memory of the writer as well as the reader. *After all, life is nothing but a collection of short stories* she thought.

It was time for Alena's sunrise to light up the dull skies of her long nights. It was a moment of self-discovery;

a flicker of hope sparked in her head, leading her to the right path. It took her forty-five years to unearth her gift, yet her passion succeeded in reaching out to her heart overnight. The uncertainty of not fully knowing her strength began to clear the way for the glimmering rays of self-awareness. She had always valued art, but she had never known until that day that she could also create it. And since she felt she did not belong anywhere in this world, she decided to create her own universe with letters and hues.

Accepting the reality of being a late bloomer in life, Alena reconciled with herself. *I know it's never too late*, she thought; *I just wish I'd started earlier.* Yet deep down inside, she was thankful she had waited for her fruit to fully ripen before picking it. *It was worth the wait.*

She took a brand-new notebook and a pen out of the drawer, and began to write — not for herself, but for her future readers, letting them explore what was inside her, the notions in her head, and the emotions in her heart. Alena was all set to unleash her suppressed feelings and guarded thoughts, to stand naked in front of her audience, with no shame of timidity or fear of insecurity. She would let her pen freely draw black and white images with words. And she went on to write the first line of her first short story.

The Truth Is One

She was distracted by the noise of the passenger train as it approached the busy streets of London. She put the amusing book in her purse, and prepared to get off. Leaving the tube station, she walked a little farther until she reached the historical building of King's College.

Her feminine high heels tapped as she walked through the corridors of the second floor of the big building. She opened the door of her office — the wooden sign distinguishing her as *Caroline Wright, Professor of Religious Studies.* The digital radio on her desk indicated that it was 8:00 AM. Dr. Wright was eager to start the winter term after the Christmas holidays, which felt much longer than two weeks.

Caroline signed in to her work email account and glanced through the messages. The Department Head had emailed regarding an anonymous complaint filed by some students of her previous class at the end of the semester. They were offended by a few of the class discussions. In a second, her enthusiasm turned into anxiety. "Another one of those! It's been a while," she sighed. She lowered her agitated head, as her hands massaged her temples. The email held a written warning that she must follow the department's curricula and present her course content objectively.

The second-year students' lecture would start in an hour. She had spent a great deal of the previous two weeks preparing this introductory presentation for the first class of the term. She was so looking forward to this lecture, but now those few lines ruined her plans. She had no time to prepare a different presentation that would satisfy her department and the few students who would never be happy. Lifting her pale face, she grabbed the mouse and began scrolling down through her older files.

She found her first lecture on religious studies from when she had first started to teach. Skimming through the slides, Caroline recalled how passionless her lectures were for her and how uninspiring for her students. *There's no way I could go back to this*, she thought. All that the PowerPoint presented were facts about some beliefs and their historical backgrounds, information anybody could find online. Most of her students had found the lectures extremely boring, but she had not received one complaint during that first year.

She jostled her way to the staff room to make some tea, and returned to her office. Holding the hot cup in her cold hands, she moved to the corner window in her office, through which she could see a tiny view of the flowing Thames. It had been raining heavily for days. Finally, the sun managed to find its way out among the dark clouds. She beheld a blurry image of herself in the glass of the window. The rays of the sun fell on her straight cherry-red hair — shinier than usual. Her sapphire earrings glowed in the morning light.

She slightly opened the window to breathe the wet air. The scent of Earl Grey somewhat soothed her troubled mind. She drew a long breath and closed the window. Turning around, she contemplated the wide board behind her desk, with quotes from many different religions and beliefs. In the centre was a quote from Hinduism: "The truth is one, but different sages call it by different names." Caroline respected Hinduism because she found it the most tolerant of all religions. In theory.

She sat down at her desk, twisting her garnet ring. She would be in the classroom in twenty minutes. She had no choice but to use her presentation as she had prepared it, yet she decided to be extra careful if the discussion got heated. If the Dean's concerns worsened, then she would decide how to proceed.

Dr. Wright entered the classroom with her well-known stern look and closed the door. The classroom was full. The students had heard that she did not allow them to enter after her; they also knew how interesting her classes were and did not want to miss any of them.

Caroline was dressed in one of her formal outfits. The graceful navy dress reflected her eyes, turning them bluer than they normally were. A fancy burgundy scarf pleasantly matched her rosy cheeks. The college-wide famous platinum necklace of the religious symbols of the world encircled her proud neck. Her simple exquisite beauty contributed to make her look like one of the classical portraits in Britain's Tate Gallery.

She began with a very quick introduction, that the first lecture was a presentation of the main topics they would be discussing in the winter term. She explained further, "I'd like to remind everyone in this room that constructive debates are encouraged, as long as everyone remains respectful of the different viewpoints. We may disagree, but we respect one another."

She turned the projector on, and the first slide of the presentation read: "Islam, Judaism, Christianity". Under Islam was Shams of Tabriz, under Judaism was Jesus of Nazareth, and under Christianity was Heresies. The first slide was intriguing enough to get the students' attention; they were wondering what sense this order could ever make to anybody.

Ismail, his thick black hair surrounding his baffled face, quietly asked, "Why is Jesus of Nazareth not logically associated with Christianity?"

"Who is Shams of Tabriz?" Jenny wondered from the other side of the classroom.

Mary, seated in the middle of the first row, asked, "Why is Mohammed not under Islam and Moses not under Judaism?" And other questions were jumping out of the students' heads.

The second slide appeared: Shams of Tabriz. The room was filled with silence. Caroline asked, "Who has heard this name before?"

"I have," answered Celine. Caroline asked her to stand up and tell the class what she knew. Confident, yet shy, Celine stood up and said, "Rumi was spiritually inspired by Shams. Together, they wrote the Forty Rules of Love."

Impressed by how succinctly she had summarised the answer, Caroline gave her the thumbs up and asked her if she knew more about Shams. Celine continued, "Shams was rejected by many fanatic Muslims, who considered his teachings blasphemy." She turned her head away and sat down.

The professor thanked Celine and added, "Shams had his own unique perspective of Islam. His whole life was a mystery, and so was his death." Caroline elaborated further about Shams of Tabriz. "Traditions say that Shams accepted people who were rejected as sinners, and rather than judge them, he inspired them to improve. Shams came to people with the message of love. He was not satisfied with the superficial interpretation of the Quran. To this day, many mainstream Imams consider Sufism a deviation from the straight path of Islam, and some look at it as heretical."

The third slide had one word: Sufism. Dr. Wright invited interested students to share what they knew. Benjamin volunteered, "Sufism is known to be the mystical approach to Islam. It is the belief that humans can reach the divine through direct personal experience with God." He stroked his thick black beard and was about to continue, but Caroline was satisfied with this brief answer. She waved a hand to stop him, and explained that they would explore Sufism in future classes. Celine insisted on clarifying that Rabia Al Adaweya was the first to introduce mysticism to Islam. "She was the single most influential woman of Islamic history," she added. Dr. Wright thanked her for sharing this information.

Caroline stayed silent for a while, going through some documents in the drawer. She could hear the humming sound in the class. "Now, after what you've heard about Shams, what has popped into your head?" Caroline asked her students.

In a second, Celine said, "Jesus of Nazareth". Smiling, Caroline jumped to the third slide. Many students were lost; they could not find a relation between Jesus and Shams.

"What do you know about Jesus?" she asked. *What a question! Who did not know Jesus?* Students thought.

One answered, "Jesus was the founder of Christianity."

Another said, "Jesus was a great teacher and a clever inspirer who gave lost people hope and restored their faith."

Mary agreed, "Jesus healed broken souls and sick bodies through forgiveness and love." She sat straight and continued, "Jesus is the Son of God who died for all humanity in order to grant them eternal life."

A student from the middle row argued, "Some people see Jesus as a mentally unstable person. Others consider him a man with supernatural powers."

"Jesus is an imaginary person. He exists only in the hearts of those who believe in him," Jenny commented, placing the tips of her soft-skinned fingers together. Jenny had moved to England from China with her parents when she was five. Her parents were keen on surrounding her with the Chinese traditions and customs, yet she also adjusted easily to the English society. She had no interest in religious studies, but she ended up in that department because she could not make it to another one. Most classes were boring to her, but she liked the heated discussions in Dr. Wright's classes.

Ismail, however, respectfully countered, "Jesus was a prophet sent by God to lead people in God's way." He adjusted the lapels of his jacket. Ismail was a gentle Muslim Pakistani who grew up in England with his moderately religious Muslim parents. It was important for him to show people, whenever he could, that Islam was not as violent as the world thought.

Benjamin wanted to share some information he learned during his research and added, "Jesus was a Rabbi who belonged to the Essenes, the Jewish mystical sect in his days, and was in constant conflict with the Pharisees." He leaned back in his seat, crossed his legs, and began to write in his notebook. He swiftly looked up and continued, "The Dead Sea scrolls have many similarities to his teachings as recorded in the Gospels."

Finally, Celine, who had her hand raised since she heard the question, was given the chance to speak: "Jesus introduced faith to his people from a new perspective. He may have shared some of the traditions of the Essenes, but he added universal dimensions to their beliefs. He restored women's dignity and respect. He came with the message of inclusion for all, instead of the literal interpretation of scriptures and the judgemental attitude." She tucked a lock of hair behind her ear and sat down.

"Thank you, Celine," said the professor. A simple, conservative smile brightened up Caroline's face and washed away her worries and fears. She nearly forgot about the tension with the department and the complaint. Nothing in the world could motivate her more than listening to her brilliant students replying to her perplexing questions with contradictory answers. Seeing most of students getting involved in the discussions inspired her to feel at ease and move on. She remembered Celine and Benjamin, whom she had taught the previous year; they usually argued opposite opinions in her classes. Celine's views usually resonated with Caroline.

Celine was an intelligent young lady who looked Asian but sounded very British; she was born and raised in England to non-religious Vietnamese parents. At the age of sixteen, she decided to start exploring all kinds of beliefs, hence her undergraduate degree in the department of religious studies. Celine was interested in spirituality while exploring the secrets of the universe.

Dr. Wright went on to the next slide that read, "Jesuism" and continued, "You may not find the word Jesuism in dictionaries. By Jesuism, we simply mean the philosophy of Jesus of Nazareth. For tens of centuries, beliefs and theories debated over many aspects that surround the controversial Jesus." Caroline clasped her arms behind her body. "Some people tried to prove that he never existed in the first place. In the midst of the endless arguments, the very essence of his message has been regrettably lost," she said.

Dr. Wright walked forward to the front row as she elaborated, "Scholars were so busy arguing about his birth and death that they missed the most important part in between — his life." Dr. Wright folded her arms. "There's no difference between those who bowed at the feet of Jesus and those who hanged him on the cross. Neither of them chose to listen to him." Caroline heard the fuss and saw, in front of her, frowning eyebrows, narrowed eyes, dropped jaws, and faces turned away, unconcerned. She whirled around, as she said, "We'll have three classes to analyse the philosophy behind Jesus' teachings."

Caroline never forgot the Anglican Church where she had grown up. Until that day, she still remembered the stories about Jesus and loved his message of salvation. She had learned early in her life that Jesus' wisdom was one thing and Christianity as a creed was another. In her youth, she had read about Buddha and his practical, positive, realistic approach to life. She was impressed by his similar concept of self-enlightenment, and noticed how, in the same way, his followers over the centuries had turned his message into a religion, and him into a god.

"Who was the founder of Christianity then, if it wasn't Jesus?" Mary asked, her freckled cheeks blushing under her puzzled green eyes.

"Very good question! Any thoughts?" Caroline encouraged her students to participate.

Celine commented, "Jesus didn't found a new religion or establish new laws. He didn't write a holy book. In fact, he was written about. Christianity as a doctrine was founded later by the writings of Saul of Tarsus, and other disciples."

"The Roman Empire made Christianity the official religion of the empire in the fourth century," from the back row, sharp-eyed Benjamin firmly argued, "that's why and how it spread all over the world." He ran his hand through his curly shoulder-length black hair.

Benjamin was also born and raised in England to strict Jewish parents, yet he was a proud atheist. In his adolescence, he had read about all religions. He had found all holy texts repetitive and boring, and concluded that the existence of the divine was not something he was interested in, as long as science had not proven it. One of the main reasons that he had chosen religious studies as his major was to prove that religions were not suitable for the twenty-first century.

"Why did the Roman Empire choose Christianity in particular to make it the religion of the Empire after a long history of their killing and persecuting Jesuists for three centuries prior?" the professor asked. "Remember that the followers of the new faith were only 10% or less of the Empire population." Caroline challenged her students, as she roamed around. The whispering sound escalated. Dr Wright advanced to her desk and searched the internet, letting students have some side conversations.

Celine wanted to share her opinion, although she seemed somewhat hesitant. In her analysis, "Jesus' disciples were also persecuted by the Romans; history clearly indicates that. Contrary to the Empire's plan to crush the new faith in its cradle, the followers increased in number, and so did the persecution against them. Finally Emperor Constantine decided to embrace the new faith and use it for his own benefit, rather than fighting it."

Dr. Wright tilted her head to one side, while listening. "This is an interesting point of view, Celine, worth considering. You are correct, only then was Jesuism turned into Christianity," Dr. Wright concluded, "as it gradually turned into rituals and dogmas, doctrines and creeds."

Benjamin's glowing eyes widened behind his glasses, as he added, "And emperors and bishops united to attain the ultimate power."

Jenny commented, "The church theologians were too busy arguing about the two natures of Jesus Christ." Her straight black bangs almost covered her narrow eyes, as she continued, "The church split."

Ismail added, "The day came when the Pope of Rome called for the Crusades, claiming it was a sacred duty to free Jerusalem." Ismail shook his head with disapproval, as he jammed his hands into his front pockets.

A vexed voice firmly interrupted, coming from the middle row. "The Crusades were a response to the persecution that the Eastern Christians suffered under the Islamic Empire rule at that time, which still happens until this day. Growing up as a Christian in the Middle East, I lived through it," Lydia said. Her olive skin sweated discomfort, as she lifted her shoulder in a half shrug. She put her curly brown locks up in a bun to cool her head off.

Isaac said, "The Crusades were no different from what is happening now with Islam and terrorism. Islam was the political movement that formed the Islamic Caliphate." Isaac tugged at his shirt collar.

Ismail's breath quickened, as the blood of his body rushed to his disturbed head. His chestnut face turned burgundy wine. He looked to Isaac and asked, "Isn't Zionism a political movement as well? In Judaism also, you can't separate religion from state."

Isaac let a sharp breath out and responded, "The Jews had suffered for centuries in Catholic Europe and Islamic Middle East, for no reason other than their ethnicity."

"And now the Palestinians are suffering," Ismail replied, lips curled with icy contempt.

"All the Jews ask for is to live with dignity and respect," Isaac interrupted. He rested his chin in his palm and looked thoughtful.

An uneven voice from the front right corner added, "On our land." Caleb Levy punched the air.

Another distressed voice coming louder from the last row interrupted scornfully, "Your land! Are you kidding me?" Mostafa Amin made a face. A chaotic, intense buzz exploded from that side of the room.

Before anyone could argue further, Caroline firmly interjected, "Time for a quiz." *Quiz! The first lecture of the term?* Students were surprised. The professor turned to the white board and wrote in big capital letters, "THE UNIVERSE". The room became soundless. She asked every student in the class to take out a blank piece of paper and pencil, and draw the first thing that came across their mind at that particular moment, and write their name on top. "You can add colours if you wish," she added, pointing at a big box of coloured pencils on her desk.

She played soft music on her laptop and gave them ten minutes to release some negative energy and calm their souls. Many students walked up to the front and picked some colours from the box. When she collected all the papers, she redistributed them in a way that every two students received each other's drawing. She chose every pair wisely. Caroline asked them to look at the picture and write a short paragraph of maximum 200 words about the drawing. She explained that every pair of students would get the same mark for their collective work.

While all the students were puzzled, Celine grinned when Caroline gave her Benjamin's drawing. She looked back at him; their eyes met. She turned her head and looked down at his drawing and started to write; her cheeks blushed behind her glasses. Benjamin had drawn a crescent with a beautiful long-haired lady sitting on it. Caroline was not surprised by Caleb's reaction when she gave him the drawing he would have to comment on. Sighing, he dropped his fist on the desk; his thick eyebrows bumped together in a scowl.

Students were given ten more minutes to write, during which Caroline walked up and down between the rows, glancing at the drawings. Her high heels struck a low note on the wooden floor, mingling in harmonious rhythm to the delicate tunes of the piano. When the quiz was over, Dr. Wright stopped the music and returned to the same slide, letting Mary speak because she had asked to add something.

Mary commented, "The history of the church has many black periods, but it should not mean that all people who serve in the church are after authority and power."

Mary was a devout Catholic; her church both satisfied and fulfilled her. She lived a simple life with her Irish family — serving and giving to whoever was in need. Caroline agreed and thanked Mary for reminding the class of this critical point; she added that generalising was never the solution.

Benjamin elaborated, "Throughout history, and in every culture, whoever seeks power and authority usually takes one of two routes — either religion or politics. The cleverest are those who combine both, and the most naïve are those who follow them."

Celine claimed, "Religions are merely human attempts in different places in the world to understand the divinity; they aren't sacred messages sent from above."

Jenny nodded. "It's enough to search how the 'sacred'," air-quoting the word as she continued, "texts of any religion were compiled to conclude that they're actually not sacred." She undid her ponytail and shook out her hair.

Celine agreed and added, "This doesn't, however, lessen their value. Those texts should be respected as part of the human heritage like literature, art, and science, but they should never be regarded as flawless or sacred. It's beneficial to examine and question them in search of the truth."

The buzzing murmurs of some students filled the classroom. "One of the problems with the world is that most people confuse faith with religion," Dr. Wright concluded, leaning forward on her desk, chin up.

She encouraged all students who disagreed to speak up and explain their point of view. Mostafa, in the last row, muttered to his friends, "There's no point in arguing with people who don't believe that holy messages were sent from God." His turquoise eyes diffused opposing energy. His voice was not loud enough for Caroline to hear, but Benjamin heard him, and watched the students in that corner for the rest of the lecture. The commotion from that corner increased. They continued muttering among themselves, yet none of them spoke to the class.

Dr. Wright felt the tension. Although she had only one slide left to finish her lecture, she decided to give them a fifteen-minute break. Mostafa rose and walked toward

Caleb at the front, and they engaged in a conversation. Benjamin was curious; he watched them from the back. He could tell that they were discussing the quiz; they had both tried their best to write good comments on each other's drawing in order to get good marks. Together they left the classroom, heading to somewhere Benjamin could not guess.

Caroline walked back to her office, wondering what could ever be offensive in educated debates. The majority of students were interactive in her classes, but every year, there had to be some who were never satisfied. She sat at her desk. Her office phone indicated a voice message. It was from the Department Head, asking to schedule a meeting with her the following morning. The tension cracked Caroline's head.

She turned to her computer and opened a folder she had made for complaints. Six subfolders had been filed by the date she had received each complaint over the years of her career as a professor. She created a new subfolder and named it *January 7th 2020*.

Her head drooped. One hand supported her chin and the other held the mouse, while she scanned through the previous complaints, reminding herself of all their similarities. *Seven complaints! There must be something wrong. Something needs to be changed,* she reflected. She recalled the challenges she had faced every time she had to justify to the department her professional goals, her tools to achieve them, and her reasons why they were pertinent. This time she was not ready to go through this. She started to doubt if it was even worth fighting for. *When will you ever give up?* she asked herself.

She began to wonder if it had been the right move to make a major career change in her early forties when she had decided to start her graduate studies in comparative religion. Yet she knew exploring other beliefs had answered many of her questions and teaching had fulfilled her needs to be challenged. Interacting with younger generations had inspired her with eye-opening perceptions. As she gained experience, she designed her lectures to be open discussions with students rather than her dictating information and asking questions. Many of her students enjoyed the engaging arguments in her classes; however, a few took offence at other students' remarks. The same obstacles had arisen from one year to the next.

Now it was impossible for her to go back to presenting meaningless and uninteresting lectures; it was equally out of the question to let her profession and reputation be destroyed. But she was sick and tired of fighting. Perhaps an alternative was to take early retirement and save face.

But where else could she ever find this incredible fulfilment that she experienced with her students? And what would she do with her time? She had not practised engineering for over a decade. She doubted if exploring fashion design was even an option now. *My teenage dream!* She gave a wry smile. Whatever her decision would be, she had to go back to the classroom and finish her lecture now. The students were waiting.

Caroline returned to class and resumed the lecture. She moved on to the next slide — Christianity and heresies — and asked students about some heresies opposed by the church. They discussed briefly the main aspects of each movement and concluded that all of them were basically arguments about Jesus' person. The next slide was about Gnosticism.

Caroline let Mary explain what she knew. "It's the position that humans were divine souls trapped in a material world created by an imperfect god. That's why the church rejected it," Mary's innocent eyes looked at the slide as she spoke.

Celine added, "The word gnosis means knowledge in Greek. The main essence of Gnosticism is that humans could reach the divine through self-enlightenment."

Benjamin added, "The church had dictated that Gnosticism was a terrible heresy, but nobody knew what it was until the Gnostic gospels were discovered in the twentieth century in Upper Egypt. Among them was the Gospel of Mary Magdalene."

Celine continued, "Mary Magdalene is portrayed as one of the leading preachers after Jesus. An inspirational female icon!"

Dr. Wright tried to draw the students' attention to compare Sufism and Gnosticism, and identify the similarities and differences between them. She told them that the last three classes of the term would be on Gnosticism. As always, Caroline encouraged students to share their thoughts.

After having reflected for a few minutes, Celine explained, "Both Sufism and Gnosticism call for finding the divine within: Sufism through the heart, Gnosticism through the mind."

"And they were both rejected by their mainstream religions," Benjamin added.

Dr. Wright pointed out the Kabbalah concept in Judaism. "It's the mystical interpretation of the Torah," she said, and told them that the last lecture would be a brief introduction to Kabbalah.

Caroline ended the class and the students were dismissed. Most of them, however, stayed in the room talking. The room was getting very noisy. Pretending to finish some paperwork in the class, she listened to their discussions. She could barely hear anything. Although curious, she had to leave.

Walking to her office, Caroline saw tiny, black-haired Celine, talking with Benjamin who seemed very tall and big compared to her. Celine came to talk to her. "I love your lectures, Dr. Wright; they're inspirational," Celine said. Caroline was surprised. How bad she needed to hear those encouraging words at that moment! Benjamin followed them, and Caroline invited both to her office. Benjamin expressed his respect and admiration for the professor and her classes.

"What were you arguing about?" asked Caroline.

"Atheism," Celine answered. A new topic for discussion was opened in the professor's office.

Benjamin respectfully explained, "I believe in what I see, hear, smell, taste, and touch. I believe in scientific discoveries and logical explanations. Death is the end of my existence." His large brown eyes smiled as he continued, "A person is but a memory; you live your entire life working to leave a good legacy for your loved ones." Caroline folded her arms and attentively listened when Benjamin continued, "A person's life is a very small contribution to the history of human achievements; you do your share to add to what people before you did, and leave it to people after you to complete. This is, in short, my philosophy of Atheism." Benjamin leaned back in his chair and lowered his head, looking at the notebook between his hands.

Caroline leaned forward on the desk. Impressed by how Benjamin explained the positive meaning of believing in nothing but the materialistic world, she replied, "Not all beliefs have to be metaphysical; even believing in nothing spiritual could have a deep philosophical sense as well. I like the way you look at it, Benjamin." Benjamin lifted his gaze to Celine.

Unable to sit still, Celine argued, "We don't see, hear, smell, taste, or touch the gentle breeze, but we know it exists because we feel it. If science can't explain something, it doesn't necessarily mean it's a myth; it could be a mystery, and science hasn't reached that far yet to explain it." Celine turned her eyes from Benjamin to Dr. Wright and continued, "If someone had told people in the fifteenth century that they would be able to hear and see someone on another continent instantly, they would have thought they were hallucinating. Sometimes, we accept a perception based on intuition, and then let logic and science take their time to explain it."

Caroline clapped her hands. "Well said, Celine. I love your take on this," she said. "Faith cannot be explained; it can only be experienced." She admired both Benjamin and Celine a great deal. Their intelligence revived Caroline's hope in the new generation.

"Unfortunately," Celine extended, "these days, Atheism has become a religion of its own, with fanatics looking down on anybody who believes in anything."

Caroline could not help getting worried that the discussion in her office could be used as evidence against her. She rose and walked to the door to peek at the hallway, as she said, "Nine times out of ten, when people dispute, they're usually talking about the very same concept but just giving it different names." Caroline sat down, feeling better that the hallway was empty.

Celine agreed, "It's wise to listen to the opposite opinion and learn about its argument. Only then will you realise that every point of view provides its own evidences and logical clues." Benjamin stared at Celine in silence, as she ran her hand through her long black hair.

"The truth is one," Caroline affirmed, pointing at the quote behind her, "but different sages call it by different names. Call it creator, evolution, destiny, big bang, first cause, universe, eternal energy, origin of spirits, redeemer of souls, beginning and end, internal voice of insight, or inner light within. They're all one thing. Name it as you wish, and live!"

Caroline picked a book from the bookshelves. The book cover was vividly coloured. She gave it to Celine. "Read this book. You'll enjoy it. It presents the history of human faith starting with polytheism, passing by monotheism and antitheism, and ending with pantheism," Caroline said. Celine and Benjamin looked at each other with enthusiasm, as if they were silently suggesting to each other that they wanted to read it together. They asked her if they could be partners for the first assignment. "I'm sure it will be one of the most interesting to read," Dr. Wright agreed.

Celine and Benjamin thanked her for her time and left. They walked from her office to the cafeteria, talking about the quiz. Benjamin laughed at Celine's drawing, but he assured her that he wrote a good comment on it. They both remembered the professor's tricky quizzes that she had used the previous year when discussions became heated in her classes. Benjamin confessed that he had tried many times to attract Celine's attention, but she always seemed to be out of reach. "Did you really?" Celine blushed. *You definitely got my attention a long time ago,* she silently admitted.

In her office, Caroline started writing a reply to the Department Head's email. Her conversation with Celine and Benjamin revealed to her that standing up for her beliefs was not in vain. The battles that she had fought paid off. Mentally too tired to think, she needed to take her mind away from her dilemma, leave everything and go home. She reviewed her reply and clicked on the send button. She rose from her seat to get ready to leave. Standing behind the glass window, she could feel the biting wind. She put on her coat, gloves and hat, and locked her office door.

On her way out, she met Dr. Guerin, who stopped her in the corridor. "Hello Caroline, Have you received my email and voice message?" asked Violette, her fluffy blond hair shining around her serious face.

"Yes," Caroline confirmed, "I've just sent you my reply."

"We need to talk. Some students say the lectures lack objectivity and are very opinionated. We talked about this last year, and the year before."

"I am objective in my classes. But I also encourage all students to share their thoughts and take part in discussions as long as they respect each other."

"That's not what they say," Violette disagreed, "they feel your classes are influential. Caroline, we're not preachers. We're scholars. It's essential to be unbiased."

"I only encourage them to dive into the deep inspirational meanings of whatever they believe in," Dr. Wright firmly defended herself, eyes crinkling.

"The college is not the right place to teach them that." Dr. Guerin tapped her foot.

"If the ultimate goal of education is not to make our world a better place — then close our schools," Caroline said, looking away.

"You're not going to change the world, Caroline. They come from different backgrounds. You can't please everyone," said Dr. Guerin, her back stiffened as she looked up to Caroline's defiant blue eyes.

"But I can, at least, point out the one essence of all beliefs to unite them," said Caroline, looking at her watch.

"You're insulting some of them. Please try to stick to the curricula suggested by the department."

"I've got to go now. Sorry, can we talk tomorrow?"

"First thing in the morning, come to my office," Violette nodded quickly.

At the cafeteria, Celine and Benjamin were discussing the rumours they had heard students gossiping about in the morning. "I can't think of any student who doesn't like her classes," Celine said, head between hands.

"The very few who stay silent all the time, perhaps," Benjamin guessed. His eyes rolled skyward.

"Who? Do you know?" Celine asked, narrow-eyed.

"I was sitting close to him, the tall blonde guy in green at the back, who was muttering all the time. I followed him going out with another student during the break and saw them talking with Dr. Guerin in her office," Benjamin revealed, "I don't know their names, but I'll find out." He blew out his cheeks.

Celine raked her fingers through her hair and puffed out her chest. "We have to support our Professor," she said.

"If things escalate," Benjamin suggested, "we'll speak to the Dean and to the President if we have to. They need to hear our side of the story."

Imprisoned by a Mirror

It was 7:00 PM, and the party had already started. They had to leave soon for the fiftieth birthday party of Scott's friend, but Gloria was still standing in front of the mirror, unsatisfied with how she looked. She had spent over three hours getting ready. Standing in the bedroom, she looked at her image in an elegant crimson dress — exhausted and sweaty.

On the bed lay strewn huge piles of countless outfits and dresses that she had tried on but would not wear. On the dresser were many makeup products, hair extensions, hair spray, skin lotions, and anti-aging creams. The garbage can was full of tissue paper, from having removed and reapplied her makeup — twice. She tried three different hair styles, but she was not happy with any of them. She stared furiously in the mirror. She was angry at herself, at her image, at people, and at the whole world.

Tired of waiting, Scott came into the room. "What on earth is all this mess? Are you ever going to be ready? We have to leave now," he railed impatiently.

She turned on him aggressively, "I'm not going anywhere."

"Excuse me? I've been waiting for hours," Scott complained.

"I don't feel like partying or seeing people," Gloria said, turning her face away.

"You look good. I like this dress on you," he said, trying to deflect her anger, "let's go, we're already late."

"I'm not going," she insisted.

Scott was not surprised, but he felt immensely frustrated. He did not want to go to the party by himself;

all his friends would be with their wives. He called his friend to apologise — they would not be coming after all. He went to the kitchen and washed the dishes, which still sat in the sink from lunch, and cleaned the counter tops. "Until when will I have to clean up after her?" he muttered, clattering pots and pans in the sink.

In her room, Gloria screamed silently, pressing her hands to her ears. She went to smoke a cigarette on the balcony to escape the irritating noise. *No matter how much I clean, it's never good enough for him anyway.* She gritted her teeth, the cigarette hanging immobile in her mouth.

He spent an hour tidying up the kitchen and the living room. He dusted their many family pictures from California, Florida, and Mexico on the fireplace. He went through piles of papers and magazines, and organised them. He vacuumed the carpet. He was not satisfied until the room was meticulously organised and completely clutter free. Then slamming the door, Scott left the house and walked to the closest Starbucks. He ordered a large black coffee and sat down to read the *New York Times.*

Gloria returned to the bedroom, pulled off the red dress, threw it on the floor, put on her pyjamas, and closed the door. She stayed in bed, gazing with enraged blue eyes at the ivory wall. Her straight golden blonde hair was badly damaged by the curling iron. Her elegant earrings lay on the floor — broken.

Will I ever get these demonic thoughts out of my head? She raged. Looking at the wall, she viewed images flickering and playing out in front of her eyes, recalling her childhood and youth. She was not even ten years old, sitting beside her cousin who was her age, when their grandmother commented on how beautiful her cousin was, how pretty her big dark eyes were, and how lovely her curly hair was, as if Gloria had not existed. Not one word of praise was said to Gloria. All she heard was the constant admiration of her cousin's beauty. Every time they visited her aunt and her grandmother, that was what she heard.

As a ten-year-old, she naively believed that she never deserved any words of praise. *I must be ugly,* she thought. She turned to her mother, wondering why she did not make her beautiful. Sadly, as childish as it sounded, this stuck in her mind beyond her childhood, accompanied her during her adolescence, her youth, grew as she matured as a woman, until that day. She still heard her grandmother's comments echoing in her ears, and she saw the shadow of her gorgeous cousin in every beautiful lady she met.

Realising that she was still awake and feeling a painful migraine that almost split her head, Gloria swallowed two extra-strength aspirin, went back to bed, and fell asleep in five seconds. The next morning, she slept in until noon. Staying in bed, she stared at the ceiling and at the opposite wall, until a reminder on her phone went off for an appointment in her calendar. The support group was meeting at 1:30 PM. She had discovered the group for women who suffered from Body Dysmorphic Disorder a few months earlier, but had been reluctant to go to any of their meetings. She had been reading about BDD. Learning about all the symptoms in detail, she easily diagnosed her own case. She knew for sure that she hated her own image in the mirror. Although she felt indifferent, she knew she wanted to go this time.

That morning she felt calmer than the previous night. Although she was too tired to be angry, she still felt bitter. She had more miserable than good days, but once in a while, she had some happier moments. She never understood why. Sometimes she was calmer and more willing to accept her belief that she was not good-looking.

Already late for the group meeting, she did not spend as much time getting ready as she normally would have. She grabbed her black sweater and jeans from her wardrobe, took a quick shower, put on her clothes, dried her hair quickly with the blow dryer, and put on her basic necessary makeup. She looked at herself in the mirror and thought, *no matter how much time I spend on my makeup or doing my hair, I'll look ugly anyway. Why even bother?*

Scott was watching TV in the living room when Gloria came in with a coffee. He was surprised that she was dressed to go out; she rarely left the house since she had resigned from her job three years earlier. He tried to figure out where she was going without asking a direct question. "You look good," he said; "it must be an important appointment." He tried to get her attention.

"It's a support group meeting. I hope it will be worth my time. I'll tell you about it when I come back," she briefly answered, looking down.

Scott was an ideal family man. A paediatrician, he dedicated half of his time to working in the hospital and the clinic, and the other half to his home. He sincerely loved Gloria, and during their first years together, his life had revolved around her. He had suggested many times that she go see a psychologist he trusted to seek professional counselling, but she was never convinced.

From Gloria's viewpoint, Scott was never good enough. She always believed that he lacked the self-confidence to seek a more beautiful lady, and that he had married her only because he did not have a better choice. A perfectionist, he drove her crazy in their daily interaction. Gloria hated his lack of self-confidence, which was why he often belittled others, but never her. Although Gloria's self-assurance was also shaky, she never put anyone down except herself and Scott.

She looked in the mirror beside the door one last time, put on her sunglasses, covered half her face with a plaid grey and black scarf, and walked to the subway station. Although it was another rainy day in New York, she took the longer way through Central Park. Holding up her umbrella with one hand and a cigarette in the other, she walked slowly. She didn't look at the amazing tulips sprouting and the wonderful daffodils coming back to life; instead, she got lost in the raindrops hitting the ground and the umbrella above her head. Her reluctant steps took her back twenty years earlier.

It was a miracle that Gloria had survived her teen years and reached her twenties. At twenty-one she was a beautiful young lady — except in her own eyes. After successfully graduating from the New York City Ballet School, she became a ballet instructor. Gloria's love for dance was equalled by her creative teaching. She developed strong friendships with colleagues at work and from the college, and she thought she could finally start to live a normal life, and accepted the reality that she was not beautiful.

She met Andrew, the brother of her best friend, Sheila. He always made her laugh, and she loved that about him, a good sense of humour being the first thing that attracted Gloria to a man. She had a secret crush on him, believing that he would never even notice her existence, especially with his attractive body and handsome eyes.

One evening, Andrew showed up at a party in place of Sheila, and told a surprised Gloria that he was her date for the night. They had a long conversation, and his interest made her glow. The following morning, the sun looked brighter to her when it shone; everything felt different to Gloria. She was over the moon. A few weeks later, Andrew accepted to work for a prestigious computer hardware corporation on the other side of the country, and left for Los Angeles. She had never seen or heard from him since.

She met Scott through a mutual friend, only two weeks after Andrew had left. Scott loved her the moment he laid eyes on her. Gloria was relieved to find someone to help her forget Andrew, but she did not love Scott; she only loved the fact that he loved her.

All the words of praise Scott gave her failed to change her self-image, or the way her eyes appraised her face. No matter how sincere he was when he told her how pretty she was, or how smart and successful she was in her career, his words could not penetrate her mind.

Gloria arrived at the New York Women's Foundation, located in a huge building in the heart of the city. She headed to the front desk, signed in, and entered the room where a small group had gathered. Somewhat late, she took a seat that was still available in the big circle arranged in the room. Most participants were already there. She looked at all the women and wondered *why are they here? They're all so much prettier than me.*

After a few minutes, the group leader entered the room and prepared the projector. When all participants were ready, she started a five minute video, followed by a brief definition of BDD which appeared on the screen and was left on during the whole session. *Body Dysmorphic Disorder is a mental disorder in which you can't stop thinking about one or more defects or flaws in your appearance — a flaw that, to others, is either minor or not observable.*

Then the facilitator started the discussion by saying, "Hello everyone, I'd like to welcome all of you. The purpose of this group is to support each other by sharing your experiences, thoughts, and stories. My name is Valerie; I've been facilitating workshops on BDD at several Women's Associations across the country for five years. I joined a support group, exactly like this one, seven years ago to seek help because I hated the way I looked."

"I am here today to listen to you," she continued, "not to speak to you. Each one of you will have an opportunity to say something about yourself. Why are you here today? What do you expect to gain? If your turn comes, and you do not feel quite ready to speak, just say 'pass'. You can also benefit just by listening to the stories of others."

Every one of the group took a turn for five to ten minutes to say something about herself. One girl said she was bullied as a child by her friend, who always made fun of her nose. Once, she was playing with her friends at school, when her friend rudely commented on her nose and how big it was, calling her a pig.

Another woman said that the way her husband treated her made her feel unattractive and unwanted. Another woman felt disgust for her fat body, and told the group how hopeless it was for her to lose weight. One woman said her mother was the main person who had instilled the thought that she was ugly in her head.

Gloria listened to all the stories the women shared about their lives until it was her turn to speak. She introduced herself, but chose not to share any personal stories. She was too worn out to speak. At the end, the leader closed the session, concluding, "Some young ladies may think they are not good-looking just because, since their childhood, they have been hearing unkind comments about how they and others look. The question should be: why do we have to compare?"

She elaborated, "Some people prefer chocolate ice cream; does this mean vanilla doesn't taste good? Like different flavours of ice cream, every girl is beautiful in her own unique way. Blonde or brunette, white or black, short or tall, skinny or chubby, they all come in different shapes and colours, yet they're all gorgeous. Don't forget that many of you are or will be mothers. You should always keep in mind Marilyn Monroe's famous quote, "All little girls should be told they're pretty..." After all, true beauty comes from within.

Marilyn Monroe's quote showed up on the screen in bold letters and stayed there; leaving the projector on, Valerie left the room. Gloria remained seated, looking motionlessly at the big screen, while the rest were collecting their belongings and getting ready to leave. Realising that the room was empty, Gloria quietly left the building.

The rain had stopped. She walked all the way to the Hudson River, and went down to stand at the bank. Observing her small image in the water, she perceived how insignificant she was. She couldn't stand looking at her reflection.

She sat down on a bench and smoked a cigarette. For the first time she felt selfish. All her life, she had always felt sorry for herself; now she felt guilty. She was confused. Was she the victim or the perpetrator? She had ruined her own life and the lives of her loved ones because she herself was broken.

It had always been about herself: her beauty, her face, her hair, her body, her clothes, and her mood. Now she found herself thinking about Belle. Gloria wondered if she gave her daughter the attention that she may have lacked. *Did I ever say something to Belle that may have shaken her self-confidence?* She panicked. Her attention gradually shifted toward Belle. *She's a teenager and needs my love and care now more than ever,* she reflected.

Gloria picked up her phone and called Belle.

"Hey, Mom. What's up?" Belle asked.

"Hello darling, I just wanted to say hi," Gloria said.

"Are you okay, Mom?" Belle asked.

"Yes, I'm okay. Where are you?" Gloria threaded a hand through her hair.

"I'm with Sarah, shopping on Broadway. We're almost done, and I'm coming home right after."

"No, don't go home. I'm here, close by. How about if you come meet me after you're done your shopping? We can go for drinks or dinner, then for a walk. It's finally stopped raining, and the sun is beautiful. I want to spend some time with you." Gloria threw the cigarette in a puddle of rainwater.

"Okay. Text me where you are, and I'll be there in thirty minutes. Bye for now."

Belle put the phone in her pocket. "I'm wondering why she wants to see me," she said. "I'll have to listen to a long lecture on my bad choice of clothes and that they won't fit my body," Belle mumbled. Sarah laughed. They walked to the subway station. Sarah took the train, and Belle continued walking.

Still sitting at the river, Gloria searched for a good café on her phone. She drew in a deep breath of fresh air, and awakened to the beauty of nature around her. She sent Belle a text with the address of the River Café where she would be waiting for her. As she opened her overly-stuffed purse to put her phone back, the oval mirror fell to the ground and shattered. Looking ahead, Gloria walked to meet her daughter, leaving the broken pieces behind.

Guilt or Grace

It was almost noon when she finished her Zumba class. The participants had noticed that she was not herself that morning. She did not talk or tell them stories during class, as usual. She did not even bring them snacks. Her eyes looked different somehow, even though her lips tried awkwardly to smile. And contrary to her habit of staying after class to socialise, she politely excused herself and quickly left after her shower in the facility change room. Her shoulder-length ash brown hair was still wet as she closed the entrance door.

The humid wind that rattled the green leaves of the tall aspen trees barely seemed to touch her, as she walked slowly through the wide lot. She often parked her vehicle far from the building to have more of a walk. Her tall curvaceous body exhaustedly moved in the snug sleeveless yellow top and the fiery red shorts. The gold V-pendant shone in the rays of the sun on her slightly-tanned skin, reflecting the brightness in her wide light-brown eyes.

Driving home, she could not help thinking about the last night she had spent with Jeffrey, when she had touched his muscular body and inhaled the scent of his hairy skin for the last time. That night, when they were alone together in the hotel room where they always met, he had regrettably announced the necessity of ending their hopeless relationship. He could not lie to his wife any longer. He was torn between his loyalty to his family and his love for Virginia, but he had made his decision. He chose his family and decided that he and Virginia would not see each other again.

She had tried with all her passion and wit to convince him that they would not be able to live without each other; at least, she knew she could not, but he did not change his mind. Only one week had passed since their last night together; and they had not even talked on the phone since then. Virginia had ached for a whole week that felt like a year to her. She did not accomplish anything meaningful. She did not want to see or talk to people. She did not go out except for her Zumba classes, where she let her distressed body leap with the musical notes.

Picking up some groceries on the way, she arrived at her Victorian house in the Riverdale neighbourhood, a ten-minute drive from the Don River to the west and Lake Ontario to the south. After putting the groceries away, she started preparing dinner. Mark and Hanna were not home; they both worked that summer to help pay for their university tuition.

Virginia marinated steak for the BBQ, peeled potatoes to cook in the oven with vegetables, and tossed up a green salad. Her phone dinged, announcing a text message. Her heart sank to the floor as she remembered Jeffrey and his non-stop messages. She knew it was not him, but every time her phone dinged, she went through the same sinking feeling. She missed him more every day.

For a whole week, all she could think about were the memories of their first meeting four years earlier — two volunteers at the community association. They had faithfully resisted the strong attraction for two years, until they finally acted on their instinctive urge, spending the past two years content and fulfilled.

After a few minutes, she thought it could have been a text from Hanna or Mark, needing something. She left everything and went to see her phone. She found a message from Alice, reminding her and Natalie of the time and place they were supposed to meet the following day. Virginia had forgotten, but they had planned for it two months earlier when they had last met.

Virginia wanted to apologise, worried if she went in this depressed mood, she might not be able to hold back her tears. After all, she could not tell them about Jeffrey. Her relationship with him was the heaviest secret in her life. But she decided to go anyway, hoping that talking to them would help her change her thoughts and feel better. She replied to Alice, confirming that she would be there.

Smelling the aroma of steak, Hanna and Mark arrived feeling hungrier than they already were. Hanna washed her hands and added dressing to the salad, while Mark checked the steak on the BBQ. Drained from the heat, Virginia went upstairs to take a quick shower to cool off physically and emotionally. In half an hour, their dinner was ready. To their surprise, Chris came home earlier than usual. "Hi Dad, you're having dinner with us!" exclaimed Hanna.

"It's Friday! Sometimes I need a break from work," Chris said. Together, they shared a good meal and enjoyed a nice family conversation about the group trip; Mark and Hanna were going to spend the weekend in a resort by the lake.

"Listen, you guys," Virginia said, "The most important thing at your age is to be extra careful of unplanned pregnancies. You're too young, and it's not a game. It's serious business." Mark and Hanna looked at each other, a little puzzled, wondering why she mentioned this now.

"Nothing will happen, Mom. Don't worry," they said. They blushed, looking down at their plates.

"They teach them this stuff at school," Chris rebuked Virginia, "you shouldn't have to repeat it every now and then. You don't want them to be paranoid."

"I can't say it enough," Virginia stubbornly insisted. "Hanna, it's your responsibility not to let yourself get pregnant, and Mark, it's your responsibility not to make a girl pregnant."

Since she had learned that she was pregnant with twins, Virginia had decided not to have more children. She was fearful of getting pregnant. Extra careful, she had been using all sorts of protection with Chris, and with Jeffrey lately. Gazing at Virginia, Chris thought that she did not look very well. She had been more positive and active until just one week earlier.

"Are you sick or coming down with something?" Chris asked.

"No. I'm just tired," Virginia replied.

"Tired? You barely did anything this whole week," Chris said, cutting the steak.

"Never mind. I'll be fine," she replied.

They ate and cleaned the table. Hanna and Mark put the leftovers in the fridge and went to their rooms. Virginia considered her relationship with Chris, as she washed the dishes. Listening to the splashing sound of water, she thought back to when they were in love. Chris was a good father to his children. An ambitious entrepreneur who owned his own Real Estate Brokerage, he spent most of the time over the years growing his business. Virginia knew he was faithful to her. She was rationally content with her marital relationship and was convinced that staying in the marriage was best for her children.

Emotionally, she was not satisfied. Their relationship was now completely tepid, although to those who knew them, they seemed a happy couple. She felt divorce was a terrible ordeal to go through; but deep down, she envied those who found the courage to divorce and were brave enough to take this final step. However, Virginia felt she had no good reason to ask for a divorce, unless she claimed adultery — her own.

Chris turned on the TV to watch a documentary about cloning. Virginia entered the family room and collapsed on the couch beside him. She watched for two minutes but found it extremely boring. She turned to Chris and said, "By the way, we're invited to Jane's wedding next month. The invitation came in the mail today." She lowered her head.

"I don't know them. I'm not going," said Chris, paying attention to what he was watching.

Virginia sighed. "But I want to go, Chris. Jane is a good friend of mine, and she would like me to be with her on her wedding day. And yes, you do know her and her family."

"You go and have fun," Chris said, squaring an ankle over one knee.

"I don't like to go alone, when all the other ladies will be with their husbands. Since the beginning of our marriage, you've always left me alone in social events like this," Virginia ranted.

"Calm down, Gina. It's not the end of the world. You know I'm not a sociable person. I don't feel comfortable in big gatherings, that's all. I don't have time. I'm busy. Take Hanna with you. She'll like it." He grabbed the remote and turned the volume up.

"I've told you a hundred times, sometimes I need you, not anyone else. But you never care. You don't even try to do anything to make me happy or to satisfy my needs." Virginia leaned back and hugged the cushion.

"I do care in my own way, but you never seem to understand or appreciate that. I care, but you're very hard to please. You live in your own world, Virginia. You need to know you're not the centre of the universe. As you think of what makes you happy, you should also think of what makes me happy. It's not just about you," Chris scolded.

Virginia went to their bedroom, which she had never deserted for seventeen years, not even when she was with Jeffrey. She was always there for Chris when he needed her sexually; she did not know whether it was out of obligation or guilt. Recently, however, Chris had not been seeking her for much — something she had hardly noticed.

Chris went to take a shower, then came out of the bathroom heading straight to her in bed. He was not very well himself, but Virginia was too preoccupied to notice. She was too sure of his being loyal to her; she never asked herself why. He slid under the fluffy purple duvet and came closer to Virginia, until his body touched hers. He started kissing her forehead, inhaling the fruity scent of her shampoo. She did not resist.

Chris said, "I need you, Gina. Stay with me. Don't ever leave me." While they were kissing, she could only taste Jeffrey's tongue. Chris embraced her, and all she could feel and smell was Jeffrey's body. Chris felt exceptionally emotional that night; he could not exactly tell why. As for Virginia, she was too lost to notice. Inattentively, she let Chris, with his excessive emotions, kiss her until he fell asleep. They were both too tired to make love.

The next morning, she got up, showered, and dried her hair quickly, eager to see her friends. She left while Chris was still in bed. She drove to Karine's, where they always met in downtown Toronto. Virginia arrived and found Alice already there waiting, and the both of them waited together for Natalie, who arrived a few minutes later. By that time, Virginia's mood was already better, and her spirit was gracefully lifted. They chatted and ordered their food. While drinking their coffee, Virginia started her curious questions as usual; she turned to Alice and asked, "Let's start with Alice. How is Mike? Are you still together?"

"Yes, we're still together. He's amazing, very kind, and understanding. We're getting married in the spring," Alice happily announced.

"Oh My God! I'm so happy and excited for you," Virginia rejoiced.

"Tell me first, how is his relationship with your daughter? This is so important," Natalie said, crossing her arms.

"Maya actually likes him very much. And his daughters are about the same age as she, so it should be fine," Alice replied.

"Just be super careful, Alice. I hear terrifying stories about men abusing their step daughters. Please be careful," Natalie murmured.

Virginia interrupted, "Oh God! Natalie, leave her alone, she deserves to be happy after years of loneliness. Yes, she'll be careful. I'm sure Alice gave a lot of thought before taking this step."

"The only reason I stayed a single mom for fifteen years was because I cared about my daughter and her feelings," said Alice quietly. "This time it's actually Maya's wish that I marry Mike."

Natalie spoke up, "Okay, you know I don't mean to scare you or hurt your feelings. All I'm saying is be careful. You two know that I have totally lost faith in men."

"I'm sorry, Natalie," said Virginia. "How is your divorce going? Is it almost over?"

Natalie grumbled, "His lawyer is a bitch. She has been dragging the case for as long as possible. Reaching an agreement on property division was ridiculously pathetic. Now, I just want it to be over. I'm never getting married again. Never!" She slammed her hand on the table.

"I'm sorry, Natalie, you're going through a tough time," Alice sighed. "It'll be over soon, and one day you'll be happy again. And never say never. You need to restore your faith in life and people."

"Easier said than done," Natalie said, looking away.

"I'm speaking from experience. Life was never fair to me," Alice said. "I went through this, and I had a baby with me, whom I had to raise by myself. I know exactly what you're talking about. It'll be over one day," Alice reassured Natalie.

Natalie turned her attention away. "And you, Virginia, what's new with you? How are the kids and Chris?"

"I'm fine. I don't have exciting stories for you. Life is good. The kids are fine. And Chris is okay," Virginia answered.

Natalie asked, "How are the Zumba classes? Do you still love it?"

"Zumba is the best thing in my life right now." Virginia leaned back in her chair.

"I was thinking of joining your class," said Alice. "How about you, Natalie? Would you like to come with me?"

"It's actually not a bad idea." Natalie pondered. "I need to release some negative energy and breathe in some positive air."

"Girls, you've made me so excited already," Virginia grinned. "Here's the phone number. Call and join. You won't regret it. We have so much fun in class. And I bring snacks every time. It's going to be terrific."

Virginia felt refreshed and in a good mood again. She realised how good life had been to her — she didn't have to go through the excruciating pain of divorce or having to raise her kids on her own. She found herself thinking of Chris and feeling very thankful for having him in her life. And for the first time, she experienced guilt; she could not understand why she was so blind to his importance in her life. She felt an urge to make it up to him for every moment she had been thinking of someone else and for all the time she had spent with another man.

She went home. Feeling energetic, she decided to clean the house. She hadn't cleaned properly for a week. She started to tidy up the entrance of the house, putting the shoes away. She picked up stuff from the family room, mopped the tiled beige floor of the kitchen, vacuumed the pistachio carpet in the family room, and did the laundry.

While she was dusting the fireplace and all the family pictures on it, she came across her father's picture. In less than a second, she remembered that it was the anniversary of his departure — thirty-five years earlier — when she was only three years old. She did not remember much about him except what her mother and her older siblings had told her. She wondered what would have been different in her life had he lived.

Virginia admired her work. She breathed the fragrance of the peonies coming from her backyard mixed with the smell of the fresh-mowed lawn. The wet clothes, billowing on the drying rack, spread the scent of the laundry detergent, which seeped in through the kitchen window. "Sometimes, we don't know how lucky we are," she murmured.

She made lasagna and stir-fried vegetables for dinner, then baked raspberry pie for dessert. At last, everything was ready and smelling delicious. Setting the table for a romantic dinner, Virginia caught wind of Chris' cologne and saw him coming down the stairs, dressed to the nines.

Lately, he had been paying attention to his looks. He had been going regularly to the gym and had lost some weight, though Virginia had been too busy to notice. She had forgotten how good-looking he was. His dark hair was nicely combed, and he was wearing contacts, so his deep brown eyes were wider than they usually appeared behind his glasses.

Puzzled, Virginia asked, "Where are you going? Dinner is ready."

"I have to go. I'm having dinner with Angela and some clients."

"Angela?" Virginia's forehead puckered.

"Yes, Angela," said Chris, preparing his briefcase.

"Oh yes, of course. Angela, your assistant. But it's the weekend. Since when do you work on weekends?" Virginia wondered.

"Since forever. Honey, what's wrong with you these days? I always have business dinners on weekends when we have clients coming from out of town. We'll show them around after dinner, as usual."

"That's too bad. I was hoping we could have some quality time together, especially since the kids are away this weekend. I spent two hours preparing a nice meal for us." She put her hands on her hips.

"You're talking as if it hasn't happened before. Gina, you know I spend most of my time at work, for work." He turned his face away.

"And with Angela," Virginia murmured. "Now I remember."

"Remember?" His brows bumped together in a scowl.

"I was too distracted, I suppose." She toyed with a lock of hair.

"Sorry about the quality time and the dinner. Eat what you can, and we'll have the leftovers tomorrow, so you don't have to cook again," he said, grabbing his car keys.

Chris left. Virginia stayed home alone. She barely ate dinner, but she had a big slice of pie. She decided to prepare snacks for next day's Zumba class. She spent time cutting fruits, and switched her brain completely off. Then she baked oatmeal cookies.

She took a warm bath. Rather than just drying her hair in ten minutes, she decided to style it, which took longer to do. She was ready for the next day and went to bed.

Staring at the ceiling fan turning too fast above her, she felt her brain become agitated. She wondered if her doubts were true. Some incidents from the near past bounced up in her memory, bringing her attention to Chris and Angela's relationship. "Maybe it's all in my head, and there's actually nothing between them except work," Virginia comforted herself. "Angela is a married woman." She burst into bitter laughter, followed by uncontrollable sobbing. She missed Jeffrey. She wished she could talk to him and tell him everything. Sitting up in her bed, she stared at her reflection in the dresser mirror as her tears rolled down her face.

She rose and walked to Chris' side of the bed. She opened the nightstand drawer. Finding nothing unusual, she closed it. *Some truths are better left unknown,* she thought. "What if it is true, though? What if Angela and Chris are in love?" If that was true, it would make everything else seem like a lie. Virginia was tortured, picturing them together. The agony was her purification. Of course, she would forgive Chris. How could she not? Yet feeling this pain was the only way Virginia could overcome the harder challenge — to forgive herself.

Hope

She was not at the hospital for work like her normal weekday. She was waiting to receive the final results for the tests which her doctor had requested for the second time to confirm his diagnosis. Christine was generally a healthy woman; she had just gone to see her doctor for her regular annual check-up. Her doctor confirmed the diagnosis and explained the case. Listening with disbelief, Christine interrupted, "I walk and exercise as much as I can."

"I'm sorry, Christine," her doctor said.

"I watch what I eat. I've lost weight recently." She gave a bitter laugh.

"We did the tests twice. Although it was obvious the first time," he explained.

"I don't drink," Christine continued.

"I understand your shock. I am sorry."

"I don't smoke," she said, eyes narrowed.

"You don't have to be a smoker to get lung cancer." He lowered his head.

"What else can a person do to avoid cancer?" Christine laughed hysterically.

"I don't know what to say. We've worked together for a long time, and you know how these things happen." He closed the file and laid it on his desk.

"But I'm fine. I feel okay. I'm not in pain." She rolled her shoulders.

"It's one of the most malignant types of cancerous tumours. I'm not surprised that there has been no pain."

"What are my options?" Christine helplessly asked.

"I want to be honest with you. There's no surgery that would benefit you. Chemotherapy and radiation are ineffective at this late stage," he explained.

Her eyes reluctantly sparkled with stubborn tears. As a nurse, she understood the case very well. With a wry smile, she asked, "How long do I have?" Her lips quivered.

"About a month or two," the doctor answered.

She stepped out of the Vancouver General Hospital, absentmindedly walked through the parking lot, passed by her car, and continued walking. It was still early in the morning. As she walked, she listened to the crunching sound of yellow and red leaves on the ground, crushed by her own feet.

Although her normal footsteps were usually fast, she walked slowly and calmly against the wind, mussing her wavy long copper hair, pulling it in all directions around her troubled head. It was chilly, but she barely felt the cold. Her mind was too preoccupied to notice anything around her. After quite a long walk, she reached English Bay; she climbed the embankment and sat on it, facing the ocean. She stared silently at the clear blue sky with her weary green eyes.

Christine sat facing the bay, which was aggressively agitated with angry waves, unlike her. She was not angry, but she was misplaced. The sound of the raging waves was harsh to her ears. She did not want to talk to any of her friends. She did not need to listen to any pointless words of sympathy, which would only add pain to her distress. She forgot about cancer and death. She only thought of Hope.

The moment she thought of her, she burst into tears that eventually grew to loud sobbing. She was thankful there were no people around — her tears flowed heavily as she sobbed even louder. "Who will care for Hope after I die?" she asked. She took Hope's photo out of her wallet and stared at it, her tears flowing down. "Why was I so stubborn?" Christine quietly howled. "Who did I think I was — the creator of destiny? Why didn't I listen to Eric? He was right." Covering her mouth she screamed, "Eric was right."

Christine was twenty-five years old, looking forward to the future with hopeful eyes, when she and Eric had married. Her dream was to have two beautiful children by the age of thirty, who would fill her time for the rest of her life. They had tried for the first two years with no results. At the beginning of the third year, she decided that they both should go see a doctor to find out the reason for the delay of pregnancy. Although the tests indicated that neither of them had major causes of infertility, the doctor suggested that she could increase her chances by a simple surgery to widen and clear her tubes.

Following the surgery, she took fertility drugs. They tried for three more years. By the fifth year, she was drained by going through the same painful disappointment every single month. That was when she suggested trying in-vitro fertilisation.

Finding this option too expensive, Eric tried to convince her to spend the money on house renovations or trips that they could both enjoy, instead of attempting what could very well not work in the end. She insisted and promised that she would budget to cover the cost. She tried in-vitro fertilisation. Twice.

She went through all the uncomfortable preparations, the medication and medical follow-up afterward, only to be disappointed again. Then losing patience, she decided to adopt. And that was when her marriage started to fall apart as she and Eric began to have serious disagreements and disputes.

It was already noon. The sun was growing more feverous over Christine's head, while she sat there not knowing what to do, where to go, or whom to talk to. She was still thinking about Hope — nothing, nobody else mattered. She recalled the day she was born, and the first time she had ever seen her angelic face and touched her silky skin. She looked back to memories of hearing her soft baby voice the first time she had uttered the word 'Mom', her first step, the first time she had a haircut, and her first day of school.

When she was younger, Hope used to ask Christine questions about when she was in her tummy, and Christine was frank in explaining that she was never in her own womb but in another woman's. She never hid the truth from Hope, deciding to tell her that she was adopted in a simple and positive way. Now Hope was nine, and Christine had to find a simple and positive way to tell her that she was going to die in a few weeks.

The salty tears, flowing from her eyes and down her cheeks, were enough to create a creek to run into the ocean and pour in it all her helplessness and vulnerability. For the first time in nine years, she regretted having adopted an innocent child, only to leave her in the world at the age of nine. "Why did I take her from her mother?" she roared.

Hours passed; she realised it was nearly two o'clock in the afternoon. She walked back as fast as she could to get her car, still parked by the hospital. Normally, Hope took the school bus home, but Christine decided to surprise her and go pick her up. She decided to spend every moment left in her life with her and start planning for Hope's life after her own death.

Driving to school, she anguished as she thought about whom she could entrust Hope's life. Her relationship with her husband had been complicated and frigid for a long time; they were a separated couple living under the same roof. Eric was against the very idea of adopting a child in the first place. Unable to predict how he would receive or perceive the news she was about to tell him, she did not know whether he would accept the huge responsibility of looking after Hope.

Then she remembered Stephanie. Christine was thirty-five when she had first met Hope's biological mother who was still pregnant at the time. Stephanie wanted to give her baby up for adoption because it was an unplanned pregnancy. Plus, she needed the money. She was a single mother who already had three kids of her own. She wished to make another woman happy by gifting her the baby that the latter could not have.

They agreed on all the details before the delivery day; the baby would be adopted by Christine and would go home with her soon after birth. It was her birth mother's wish to stay out of her life. Stephanie felt it would be emotionally torturous to watch her child growing up away from her with another woman. She only left her email address with Christine in case there was an important legal issue regarding the adoption documents. And she was happy to occasionally receive pictures of her daughter which Christine sent.

Christine thought of contacting Stephanie, but she was not sure how she would respond to the news. *Is it even wise to let her know?* Christine doubted. It had been years since Christine had sent her Hope's photo at age two, to which Stephanie had never replied. Christine was not even sure she still had her email address.

Her brain was fully crowded with many scary thoughts until she found herself in front of the school. She hurried to meet Hope before she got on the bus. Surprised and happy, Hope came running to her, and they hopped in the car. Hope enjoyed the car ride, looking at the tall trees and the falling yellow leaves. She told her mother in great detail what happened that day at school. Christine decided to take her to their favourite restaurant that had many good choices in their kids' menu.

While they were eating, Christine looked at her daughter's innocent eyes. She wanted to start the important conversation, but looking at Hope rendered her weaker than she expected. How could she start? What would she say? Christine collected all her strength to contain her ache.

Hope said, "Thank you, Mom. You're the best."

"You're welcome, sweetie."

"I wish you could pick me up every day." Hope sipped her chocolate milk.

"I wish I could, too, honey. You're so beautiful." Christine sliced Hope's pizza.

"Mom, you're my best friend," Hope said.

"How about Dad?" Christine asked.

"I love Dad, too; sometimes he's fun," Hope smiled.

"Yeah, of course. Daddy is fun." Christine rubbed her forehead.

"But you do everything with me, Mom." Hope took a bite from her pizza.

"Do you remember Stephanie?" Christine asked, rubbing hands.

"Stephanie?" Hope tilted her head to one side.

"Yes." Christine nodded.

"Who is Stephanie?" Hope asked.

"The woman who gave birth to you. Remember when I showed you her picture?"

"Oh yes, yes, Stephanie. Yes, now I remember. What happened to her?" Hope asked.

"Nothing. Nothing happened to her. I hope," Christine answered. "Would you like to meet her?" she asked Hope.

"No. I don't know her." Hope answered, chewing on a piece of pepperoni.

"I was thinking of contacting her. Maybe we can get together, if she's cool with that."

"Why?" Hope wondered.

"Why not?" Christine scratched her nose.

"I remember you told me that she lived far away in another province."

"Yes, but she may be in town soon. I thought it would be nice to meet her," Christine stuttered.

"Okay. Can we go see a movie together? It's been a while since we last did."

"For sure. Which movie would you like to see?" Christine grinned.

"*Beauty and the Beast,*" Hope suggested.

"Okay. *Beauty and the Beast.* Let me find out which theatre is playing it."

Thus, the conversation went in another direction, contrary to Christine's plan, and gradually she lost the courage to introduce the subject. While they were having their dinner, Christine gazed at every inch of Hope's face and body, not believing that she would not live to see this little green fruit ripen and taste so sweet.

As they walked to the car, Christine took Hope into her arms in a tight embrace, her suppressed tears overflowing her burning eyes when Hope could not see her face. She managed to wipe most of her tears, but the little girl was too sensitive and intelligent not to feel there was something unusual about her mother.

They arrived home, but Eric was not yet there. Christine went directly to her laptop and spent over an hour looking through her sent emails, searching for Stephanie's email address. Then she remembered that her last email to Stephanie was sent from another email account.

When she tried to recover her old email account, it was impossible to reactivate it. Even though she was not sure of the spelling of Stephanie's last name, she googled many probabilities finding many women with that name but not the one she was looking for.

She thought she might find the right spelling on the legal adoption papers that she kept with all her important documents. It was a challenge for Christine to remember the places she normally kept important documents, never mind going through them all. They could be anywhere in the house.

She looked all over the place — in her desk drawers, her closet, her old purses, her briefcase. She even looked in the kitchen drawers. At last, she found them, but was disappointed to see that she had already tried the right spelling of the last name on Google.

Eric finally arrived; he had eaten out, as usual. An IT specialist for a big corporation, Eric spent most of his time out of the house. He was not very enthusiastic about work. It was more an excuse for him to stay away from home, where he felt he was nobody important after Hope had entered it against his will. If not at work, he was with friends, playing billiards. Most of the people he spent time with were single.

He had affairs that did not last long. Feeling neglected by Christine, who gave all her attention to Hope, he had sought affection elsewhere. But he was rarely satisfied. A heavy smoker, he was negligent of his health. It was he who needed someone to take care of him. Christine had talked to him many times about taking good care of himself and paying attention to his health, until she finally gave up and decided to let him live his life the way he chose.

As Hope grew, Eric gradually got used to her presence in the house. Still, he barely spent time with her; it was partially his resentment at Christine that prevented him from developing a good relationship with Hope. For years, he could not get over the fact that she had adopted her against his will. And he was equally angry at himself for even signing the legal adoption agreement under pressure from Christine.

Christine waited until Hope went to bed and asked Eric if they could talk. It had been a long time since they sat down to have a conversation. Although he knew about her recent medical tests and doctor's appointments, the last thing he could possibly imagine was what Christine was about to tell him now. Telling the news to Eric was far easier for Christine than to Hope. Straight to the point, she said, "I've received all the test results that the doctor requested."

"And?" He leaned back in his chair.

"They all confirm his diagnosis. Lung cancer." Christine looked down at her own hands.

"When will you start chemotherapy?" Eric asked.

"No chemotherapy or radiation or surgery can do anything. It's pretty much all over my lungs and other parts of my body," she calmly answered.

"How is that possible? Do you have pain?" Eric rubbed his chin.

"No, I don't. But I will. The pain will start soon in a matter of days. I will live on morphine until…"

"What?" Eric froze up.

"I have two months to live. More or less. The problem now is Hope," Christine said.

"What's wrong with Hope?" Eric did not know where to look.

"She's fine. It's just that after I'm gone, who will take care of her?"

"Hope?" Eric said. Blood escaped his face, turning it as pale as a white China plate.

"I've tried everything to locate Stephanie, her mother, but I can't find her anywhere. I lost her email address."

"Why Stephanie?" Eric asked.

"Who, then?" Christine hinted.

"Well, I don't think she'd be willing to take her back after all these years." His shoulders sagged.

"But at least she has a right to know. After all, it's her daughter. Don't you think?"

"I don't know." He pinched the bridge of his nose.

"My last resort is the hospital where she delivered Hope. I'm going tomorrow to ask. They may have a phone number for her, an address, or something."

"But why? Stephanie has never been a part of Hope's life, and that was her own wish. How can you bring her back into her life now?" Eric argued, showing his concern.

"I'm desperate. I think she needs to know. And then the decision is hers," Christine insisted, turning her face away.

Having nothing more to say and finding no response from Eric, Christine said, "Good night," and went to bed.

Eric stayed still on the chair, unable to move one limb of his body. The shock hit him like a flash of lightning, leaving him unable to blink, looking at nothing, lost in the void. Every single word she had said to him was repeating itself in his baffled head.

It felt as if someone had pushed the off button; his brain could not function. It was as if a huge dark cloud had settled in front of his eyes, he could see nothing. He was not sure if he was still breathing. Many questions were screaming in his ears. *How could she go that fast? How could this be happening?* "What if Stephanie decides to take Hope back?" Eric asked. "Am I going to lose both of them?" he hopelessly murmured, staring at a big picture on the wall of Christine and Hope.

Eric stayed on the chair all night long, but he did not sleep one minute. The next morning, he was still on the chair when Christine prepared breakfast for Hope. After breakfast, Hope went in the car and waited for her mother, as Eric tried changing Christine's mind regarding telling Stephanie.

Confused, Christine asked, "Why don't you want Stephanie to know?"

"I told you last night." His hands tightened into fists.

"I don't understand." She shoved her hands in her pockets.

"This would be so unfair to Hope, to lose you and the life she has had since she was born at the same time. This can ruin her life. She doesn't even know Stephanie," Eric yelled.

"Since when do you care about Hope?" heartbroken, Christine wondered.

Eric did not answer. Christine left. He cared, but he was too ashamed to voice it to her. *I've been selfish for nine years. How could I punish her for wanting to be a mother?* He slammed his hand on the table. He grabbed his half full pack of cigarettes and threw it in the garbage. He knew she would doubt that he could be the right person for that task. But he did not want to lose Hope. He recalled the few times he took her to the park when she was younger, and when he once read her a story.

He wanted Christine to know that he would be a good father to Hope. But he had very little time to prove it. It was important for him to make Christine believe that Hope would be taken care of. He went to his laptop and started searching on the internet.

Christine and Hope arrived at the clinic. After a long wait, during which Christine was praying from the bottom of her heart that she would find any trace to Stephanie, they were called to see the nurse. Sympathising with Christine's desperation, the nurse asked, "How long ago was the delivery?"

Christine answered, "Nine years."

The nurse explained, "I'm sorry. Our retention policy is to keep records only for seven years." Christine's last tiny piece of hope shattered.

Christine was devastated. She did not know where to go. She did not have a sister or a brother to leave Hope with, and her mother was an old lady who lived in a nursing home. Every time Christine looked into Hope's eyes, the same question — still without an answer — pierced her heart. She wished she could ask Eric how he felt about being the person to be there for Hope, but she was too scared. Her head felt like it would explode.

They left the clinic and saw Eric, who was walking toward the building. Shocked when she saw him, Christine walked ahead pretending she was alright. When

Hope saw Eric looking at her with open arms, she ran to him. Hiding her moist eyes behind the sunglasses, Christine walked in silence, but Eric and Hope could feel her anguish before they could see her tears. Eric offered to drive, and Christine sat beside him. She stared at the bare autumn trees.

Eric breathed a sigh of relief when Hope told him they found no trace of Stephanie. "I'm inviting you to lunch at the Boat House seafood restaurant by the water," he said. Christine looked at him, confused. Her brain was unable to reach any conclusions; she refused to think of anything that might give her false hope. He gave Hope an envelope and asked her to open it.

"Oh my God," Hope screamed joyfully, "three tickets to Disney World for a whole week!"

"Yup, just booked them online this morning after you'd left. We're leaving on Sunday." Eric's smile revived Christine's decaying eyes. They had no time for tears.

Between Two Streams

Her moans interrupted the muteness of the room, as the dawn erased the blindness of the night. In the extended communities of mud houses, south of the bountiful Eastern River, her soft cries of pleasure flew out of the square window and soared to the ether. She lay on the wide step, as he passionately made love to her. His caresses released the milky juice, welling from between her voluptuous thighs, and gratifying his thirst.

The room was silent once more. She waved a hand to him to stop. She did not feel comfortable going further for complete penetration. "Perhaps next time," she said, giving him a bunch of green olives in a small clay pot.

"Thank you, my lady." He gratefully bowed and left. Kisharat would definitely call that fellow again. He knew how to gift her joy. She could not remember his name, but she was certain where to find him again — working in the quarry.

She fastened the short skirt around her waist and walked out to her brother's room. She was eager to speak with Ansarin, but he had not returned yet. Distracted, she walked to the river to wash herself. As she paced, her breasts felt heavier and fuller. *When was the last time my holy blood flowed?* Kisharat wondered, as she left the district and reached the waterway. Ansarin was not anywhere in the community.

The tender sun sent its warm rays over the land of the two rivers. The water was pristine, and the wind was serene. Some ladies were bathing, but she did not care to engage in conversation with them. She walked farther until she found a quiet spot. She took off her garment and looked at herself in the water. Her reflection showed that her belly was growing bigger. She delighted in the warm water, and as her body floated, her eyes gazed at a few patches of clouds. Kisharat finished her bath, letting the sun dry her body and hair, while her brain was still absorbed in the mysterious disappearance of her brother.

On her way back, she saluted sisters planting in the verdurous fields of wheat and barley, which spread vastly until they met the azure sky. She sniffed the goodness of the generous soil. The green leaves of the countless trees fluttered with the smooth current of air. The figs and pomegranates ripened, and their aroma was enough to satisfy a hungry stomach. As she walked slowly, Kisharat heard the echoes of brothers, carving stones for building and unearthing gems for jewellery. Farther on the horizon, more brothers scattered around the territory to protect against vicious animals and invaders.

Kisharat returned to the community, her brother still nowhere to be found. She went to her room and got dressed for the commemoration. As she entered the house of worship, she inclined her head to pay respect to Goddess Lilitha. Kisharat said a faithful prayer that Ansarin return. The last time she had talked to him many sunrises earlier, he had expressed interest in exploring other parts of the land. She had not seen him since.

The High Priestess directed five priestesses, preparing the girl of the week to offer her first sacred blood at the Shrine. They recited prayers for the communities around the rivers and supplications for Lilitha to bless their lands and the wombs of all female creatures. The priestesses braided the bride's long mane, decorating the thick braids with coral and turquoise beads. They poured scented oil made from consecrated herbs on her bare skin, and placed her naked juvenile body in front of the Sanctuary. Spreading her youthful limbs, the girl let the divine blood stream from her internal spring of life.

"O Glorified Lilitha, who gave up abundance for freedom, and walked the fearsome path alone through the dark wilderness, groping for knowledge! You who conceived all things with love, please accept this blood of life and protect your children from the demons," Mother Shetarot prayed. Three lines of deaconesses on each side of the Shrine sang hymns of rejoice, as they played their musical instruments and danced in their flowing white robes to the rhythm. The immortal serpents embraced the girl's body, swirling to the tunes. The pond of purity was full of immaculate lotus flowers, floating around in circles.

After the ceremony was over, the High Priestess gave a sermon on the rising estranged teachings against Goddess Lilitha, coming from the West. "Those people," Mother Shetarot declared, "are going astray. They've deviated from the straight path of our mothers." Prophetess Shetarot went on to explain how the foreign beliefs stripped the fertile females of their holiness by claiming that they were unable to reproduce on their own. "They don't know the truth," she said, her arms spread wide.

"They kill animals and birds, our companions and helpers, to eat them and offer them as sacrifices to their gods. Some tribes still insist on the ancient traditions of offering human sacrifices. They offer the blood of death; we offer the blood of life. They cut down trees — our source of nutrition and medication — to make into boats and chariots. They call for aggression and war; we call for security and peace." Mother Shetarot worshipped Lilitha, praised the blessed serpents, and ended her preaching.

During the ritual, Kisharat hardly paid attention to anything except for the speech of the High Priestess at the end. She recalled her last conversation with Ansarin, when he had talked about strange concepts she had never heard of until that day, during Mother Shetarot's sermon. Kisharat begged Goddess Lilitha to protect Ansarin wherever he was.

She headed to the big house in the centre of the community, the house of the head of the tribe. "Mother, may I come in," Kisharat bowed as her great-grandmother waved to her to enter. The old lady sat on the thick colourful straw mat, covering the built-in-the-wall seat. Her silver braids covered her back and shoulders, and many beaded necklaces of all colours encircled her wrinkled neck. Her small dry breasts hung above her stomach. Kisharat advanced and kissed her great-grandmother's forehead and hand. "Good day, Mother. May our Goddess keep you for the community!" She sat down beside the respectable lady and said, "I have good news, Mother. I'm carrying an infant," Kisharat rejoiced.

Nari stretched her lips in a wide smile, and her eyes sparkled with tears of joy. "Oh Kisharat, Goddess poured Her divine spirit on you to add one more member to our big family," Nari said.

Kisharat decided to ask her great-grandmother about Ansarin. The subject caused Nari's face to crinkle up with disappointment. "Your mother's son has not been seen for days. No one knows where he is, or when he will return," Nari said, brows knitted in a frown. "He may not return!"

Kisharat slapped her chest. "Who will raise my child with me then?"

Disoriented, Kisharat left to her room after she had paid respect to the old woman. She missed Ansarin; she could not wait to tell him the good news. But he was not there to share this moment with her. Ansarin's absence turned Kisharat's delight to distress that weighed on her all afternoon. Her body was too heavy to rise from her sleeping step. She did not go to the house of learning for the art group, where the sisters practised painting and writing. When it was dinner time, she reluctantly pushed herself to go out and eat with the family. All the sisters congratulated her. She ate, although she could think of nothing but when her brother would return, or if he ever would.

South of the vigorous Western River sat Bramohim ruminating by the water. He contemplated the West, where the sun was about to set and disappear. His absorbed eyes glanced at the horizon. *There is no end to this land that I can see*, he thought. He leaned back against the trunk of a tall palm tree and lifted his eyes up to the sky. The clouds moved with the wind as fast as the water in the stream.

"Are you still talking to yourself Bramohim?" His brother interrupted his train of thought.

"I was not talking to myself nor to anybody," Bramohim replied, looking away.

"Nobody believes what you say," Salomin bent down and said. "All men, who had come from the neighbouring communities to listen to you, left and went back to their mothers' land."

Battling discouraging thoughts, Bramohim declared, "They don't know their value or their power." He picked a date from the ground and munched a bite, as he continued, "They live in a lie, and they sadly believe it."

Salomin squatted beside him and spoke softly, "What are you trying to achieve, Mother's son?"

"We men deserve to know who our children are," Bramohim yelled, "and to have them named after us. To maintain genealogies, one woman must never be with more than one man. If she does, she should be punished," he growled.

"No one understands what you say." Salomin shook his head and continued, "Men are barren creatures. On our own, we would die off." Salomin slapped his two palms against each other.

"Men are the source of all offspring; without us, women can't give birth to anyone. Science knows this," Bramohim raged.

"Where did you learn this nonsense — this science?" Salomin wondered and went on, "Women are the life givers." Frustration wrinkled his forehead. He had heard Bramohim teach these unusual notions many times but still could not comprehend them. "How can we survive without our Mothers and Mother's daughters? They own all the lands; we just work for our food and shelter," Salomin wondered, turning his distressed face away.

"We don't need to work for them," Bramohim said, stroking his long grey beard.

"We were never taught how to plant. What can we eat?" Salomin asked, one hand clasping the opposite wrist.

"Follow me to the land in the West by the sea," Bramohim beseeched his brother; "we'll have our pastures. We'll grow our cattle to slaughter and eat."

"Kill animals and eat them! Have you gone mad?" Salomin's nose crinkled and his lips curled with disgust.

What Bramohim said perplexed Salomin, as it had bewildered all men who had gathered around him for days, but finally decided to leave. "Why would we leave our mothers' land and go to a foreign region, inhabited by other people? They'll destroy us," Salomin said.

"We'll fight them, and we'll win," Bramohim shouted as he hit the ground with his cane.

"I've heard this word 'father' that you keep repeating, from people in the North," Salomin said; "they worship goddesses and gods."

"There is only one God. He is the father of all of us," Bramohim proclaimed, letting out an exasperated sigh. "The practices of the mothers are infidelity. Goddess Lilitha is the devil. Women can't rule or teach; they must obey in silence. What they call the holy blood of life is impure and defiled! The serpents are wicked and evil," Bramohim roared. His voice was as loud as thunder. He rose, leaning on his staff.

"No one believes you," Salomin mocked him, "Nobody is going with you anywhere." Salomin's hands tightened into fists.

"I'm leaving alone then," Bramohim said, as he walked away from the river.

Salomin rose and went to the tent where Sarayshot had stayed behind. There were big totes at the entrance. "What are you doing?" Salomin panicked.

"I'm packing," she said, tripping over her long garment.

"What are you wearing, Mother's daughter? Why are you all covered up like that? Where are you going with him?" Salomin lifted his shoulder in a half shrug.

"I don't know where we're going," Sarayshot answered, "but I trust him."

"You too have gone mad!" Salomin said.

"I have nothing to tie me to a community that doesn't respect me because I'm not a mother," Sarayshot said in a bitter tone. Her face was sweating from discomfort under the long scarf which Bramohim had commanded her to cover her head with.

Salomin left her in the tent and walked to the farms, puzzled by Bramohim's notions, but too anxious to let him go away alone. Sarayshot continued putting away some tools and containers in big pouches. At a distance, Bramohim walked back to the tent as the sun set. He was determined to depart the following day to explore the far land in the West.

Darkness surrounded the community by the Eastern River, which was in deep slumber. The silver moon provided some frail light for Kisharat to leave the room and sit at her doorstep. The rhythmic trills of crickets in the rice fields sounded shrill in the midst of silence. Kisharat failed to get Ansarin out of her head or stop herself from worrying about her future child. It was her brother's responsibility to raise the baby with her. In her trouble, she invoked Lilitha to grant her peace and reassurance. "O Mother of Mothers, Queen of Earth, show me a sign to comfort my troubled heart," she pleaded, wrapping her arms around herself.

Her tearful eyes caught a glimpse of a small shadow coming from afar. Fatigued, Ansarin paced slowly toward the outskirts of the community; he had walked for days on a long journey from the Western River. His head was crowded with many contradictory conceptions, some he had been raised with, and some he had just discovered. In the light of what he had perceived, he felt all his beliefs collapse. He wished he could unlearn what he now knew. He longed for some comfort from his sister. He would explain everything to her.

Kisharat thought her eyes deceived her, but when he came nearer, she realised it was him. She breathed a sigh of relief. "Thank you Mother Lilitha!" she prayed. As he approached closer, she said, "Ansarin, thank Goddess you're back. I've been praying all day, asking Her to protect you during your long journey." She held him tight and said, "I'm with a child, Ansarin. We'll have one more member in our family." She ran her hand through his long hair and continued, "Don't ever leave me again, please."

Ansarin was too worn out to speak, too exhausted to stand. He went in her room and sat down on the step. She brought him some water to drink. After some silence, he said, "I wonder who the child's father is." He gave a wry smile and leaned back against the wall, gazing at the thatch roof.

"Father!" Kisharat's eyes narrowed. "Where did you learn this vocabulary?" She let a long breath out, as her hand softly touched her abdomen. "What's wrong with you, Ansarin? I'm the mother of the child. It will belong to the family of Nari, and the tribe of Seret, our great-great-grandmother. This child is the spirit of Goddess and a part of me."

"Kisharat," Ansarin said, "every child needs a mother and a father to be created. We've been wrong all along." He shook his head, looking down at the clay jug of water between his hands. "The good soil cannot produce a plant without the seed," he mumbled, blowing out his cheeks. He left her room and walked to his own. Kisharat ran after him. "Why did you come back then?" She clapped her hands on her hips, arms crooked like bowl handles.

"I'm leaving in the morning," he said, "I came to collect my belongings. Come with me, Kisharat." He maintained eye contact.

Kisharat sobbed. "Are you going back to those people who want to destroy Lilitha? She has been so good to us and to our mothers since forever." Her two hands slapped her own cheeks.

"No, I'm not going back to them," Ansarin said; "those teachings didn't appeal to me. They've gone to the other extreme." Ansarin turned around and walked ahead.

"Where are you going then?" Kisharat asked, clinging to his arm.

"I am going North in between the two streams," Ansarin revealed. He waited, hoping Kisharat would say something, but she did not. He headed to his room.

Kisharat found herself standing alone in the bleak, hushed night. She wended her way across the community to her room. She observed the dark meadows through the square window, facing the North. As the pink sunrise emerged from the East and the powerful wind blew in the blue sky from the West, she contemplated plants, birds, animals, and people moving around. And she made her decision.

Everything in nature came in female and male. *Why would the Divine be any different?* "Mother. Father. Mother. Father," she repeated the word she had always known and the new one she had just learned, while she packed her belongings.

Bitter Melodies

She finished her last thirty-minute lesson of the day, and accompanied the little girl to the door. It was three o'clock in the afternoon — time to cook dinner before Sébastien arrived from work. She played one of her classical music CDs that were neatly piled beside the CD player on the corner table in the living room and headed toward the kitchen.

She started to prepare *blanquette de veau*; she knew he loved it. She wanted to make it up to him for having been so busy with her violin lessons lately. The aroma of the veal with the vegetables coming out of the oven filled every room of the orderly house. The phone rang as she was setting the table for dinner. "Hello," she answered.

"Hi honey, I'm sorry. I won't be home for dinner tonight," Sébastien apologised. "You go ahead and eat."

"Again!" she reproved.

"I'm sorry. I have to finish something very important at work."

Disappointed, she gloomily cleared the table and put the food in the fridge. It had been two weeks since he had started to act strangely. The first few days, she was too busy to notice. But later, his absence was obvious. Taken by the obscure tunes of the third symphony of Louis Vierne, she peeked through the kitchen window at the quiet streets. The sparkling Christmas lights on the houses brightened up the bleak night.

Marguerite went to the violin room. She could spend hours playing musical notes on her cherished violin. The melodies took her to another realm of soothing sounds. She blamed herself for having been too busy in the last few months with her students. She was getting requests from many parents in the neighbourhood to teach their children, and she could never say no to that. Her reputation as a passionate music teacher spread in the schools and communities.

An hour passed, and Sébastien was not home yet. She put her violin back on the stand and walked to the living room. Classical paintings covered the ivory walls, and the room was elegantly furnished with antiques. Her home seemed like a room in the Louvre Museum. Pouring herself a glass of wine, she sat down.

She took a couple of photo albums from a drawer of the coffee table and looked at each photo. Marguerite and Sébastien loved to spend their time exploring the world. Many trips were relived through those pictures. The other album was their wedding and honeymoon; this one drew a nostalgic smile on her face. Her hair was much longer; she was a lot thinner, and he had much thicker hair back then. Their wedding was simple and intimate.

There were honeymoon photos on Santorini, the romantic island in the Mediterranean. She flipped through pictures of exquisite white houses by the azure sea. Recalling their sweet memories, she finished the whole wine bottle. Her head felt heavy. She put the albums back and went to bed. She fell asleep before he was home.

Marguerite and Sébastien had been married for nearly twenty years, and they were still in love. Among three friends, she was the happily married one. Only a harmonious match could persist over so many years. They were similar enough to make life steadily comfortable, and different enough to keep it exciting and lively.

At first Marguerite had decided to become a home-maker, dedicating her life to her home and family. Later, her passion for music and love for violin had offered a good opportunity for her to teach violin lessons at home. She loved being a music teacher, especially for young children. She felt blessed to spend most of her time with them, listening to their inspiring stories. Working from home suited her quiet personality.

The next morning, groggy from the effect of wine, she slept in until 8:30 AM. When she looked for Sébastien, she realised he had already left. Marguerite stayed in bed lacking any motivation to get up. She only had two lessons that day, one following the other, and they were not until one o'clock in the afternoon.

Picking up the phone, she called Brigitte. "What's up?" Brigitte asked, noticing that Marguerite's voice was not normal.

"Sébastien," Marguerite answered, in a glum tone.

"What happened? Is he alright?" Brigitte asked with concern.

"He's not himself." Marguerite's breath quickened. "He's barely home. He doesn't talk to me or tell me anything about his day," said Marguerite, biting her nails.

"But we were together less than a month ago, and he was perfectly normal," Brigitte recalled.

"It all started when he asked me to go on a trip to Greece two weeks ago," Marguerite sighed, "but I said I couldn't because of my violin lessons. It was on very short notice. I couldn't cancel twenty lessons just like that. I just suggested that we plan ahead, as we always do."

"Did you ask him why he was in a rush for this trip?" Brigitte asked.

"Yes, I did. He said it was a good time for him to take some days off from work. And two days later, all of a sudden, he became too busy at work to come home for dinner," Marguerite blurted, rolling her eyes.

"Have you talked since?" Brigitte wondered.

"No. He's avoiding me. He's out most of the time, claiming he's busy at work. And when he comes home, he pretends to be too tired to speak." Marguerite tossed her hair.

"You have to talk, Marguerite. I'm worried about you."

"I'm worried about him." Marguerite chewed on a cuticle.

"Well then, that's why you have to talk to him."

"I'm scared. What if there's another woman?" Marguerite twisted the wedding ring on her finger.

"Another woman! What's wrong with you, Marguerite?" Brigitte denounced.

"Why not? How can you explain why he's late every other night? What if he's not in love with me any longer? I wouldn't be able to handle it," said Marguerite, her left hand trembling over her eyes. "He deserves to be a father. I've been so selfish," Marguerite cried.

In the fifth year of their marriage, their first baby had died in her womb hours before birth. Marguerite's uterus had been damaged beyond repair leaving the doctor no choice but to remove it. With immense sadness and heartache, she had accepted the reality that she would never be a mother. She often reminded herself to count her blessings, including those in disguise. Marguerite considered Sébastien her only child and her whole family. Yet, at times, she battled the insecure feeling that one day he might leave her in quest of fatherhood.

"Marguerite, please don't jump to conclusions," Brigitte said. "A relationship doesn't start suddenly like this. If he's in love with another woman, why did he want to go on a trip with you?"

"Maybe that was what he wanted to tell me during the trip." Marguerite slapped her forehead.

"Wait until you talk. You have no reason to worry. I have a feeling he has a serious problem at work or with money, and he doesn't want to worry you, knowing how anxious you always get." Brigitte tried to calm her down.

"I'm unable to think straight, Brigitte. I'm confused. I can't believe this is happening." Marguerite bit her upper lip.

"Marguerite, listen to me. You tell Sébastien that you feel like going out for dinner tonight. You will eat out and talk. Tonight. Alright?"

After talking with Brigitte, Marguerite felt determined that she would do exactly as they decided. She got up and showered. She was hungry; she had not eaten dinner the previous night. She went to the kitchen and made coffee and two croissants with butter and honey. Trying to keep her mind busy, she flipped through *Le Monde*. An hour later, she made toast with Swiss cheese and ham, to go with another cup of coffee. The doorbell rang; it was time to start her lesson. An hour passed, and the two lessons were over.

She called his phone but received no answer. By then, her fear had intensified, and her doubts were becoming certainties. That time of the day he was normally at the office, but she had a feeling he was not. She could not let it go; unlike before, now she wanted to confront him. "Yes, I was too busy with my music lessons; so, what?" she whispered. Without thinking twice, she texted him a crisp message, saying that she had already booked a table for two at La Rivière restaurant and she would be waiting for him at 7:00 PM.

When he first received the text, Sébastien was reluctant to reply, let alone accept the invitation. He had left the house that morning, not knowing where to go; all he needed was to stay away from all this. He was not at work. She was right. Disoriented, he drove in circles until he ended up at a café. He drank coffee, staring at people walking down the street from behind the glass window. He walked to a small store where he purchased a pack of cigarettes. Although he had quit smoking five years earlier, he smoked half of the pack, sitting on a bench in front of the store. Having nowhere to go, he then went to work.

Marguerite waited impatiently for his answer to her text. Her imagination went wild. She could see him with another woman in bed and hear their sounds. It was torturous. She was so distressed that she could not find comfort even in her violin. She checked her phone messages every minute. Unable to wait any longer, she called his mobile phone again and received no answer.

Meanwhile, after considering all his options, Sébastien decided to answer her message and let her know he would be there waiting for her. He figured it might be the long-awaited opportunity that he had been looking for.

Marguerite was crying and waiting in bed when her phone vibrated, announcing a new text message from Sébastien. Jumping out of bed, she started to get ready. She stood in front of her wardrobe for about ten minutes, trying to make up her mind on which dress to wear. She picked a dress he had bought her a few years earlier, but when she put it on, it was too tight. Disappointed that she had gained weight, she finally decided to wear her burgundy outfit. An hour had passed, and she was still sitting in front of the mirror, staring at the reflection of an aging lady in a wombless body. *I'm sure he's met a prettier and sexier woman,* she thought.

The burgundy reflected in her grey eyes turning them into a mesmerising colour that had not yet been named. Her straight shoulder-length black hair gleamed like the night sky. The pearl jewellery set she wore — the first wedding anniversary gift from him — shone glamourously on her innocent round face. She blamed herself again, agonising that she could be the reason she had lost him.

She arrived on time at the restaurant, but he was not there. She was seated at a table for two that she had booked. She waited anxiously, but not for long. Five minutes later, she heard his sweet *bonjour* coming softly from behind her ears. He approached, kissing her on her left cheek, apologising for being late and holding a bunch of white daisies in his hand. He loved daisies of all flowers because they carried her name, and he chose white ones, resembling her pure heart.

Immediately she stood up, turned around, held his face gently with her delicate hands, and kissed his lips. "I miss you. We haven't talked for a while," she said, looking up through her lashes.

"I know. I've been busy," he replied, as he sat down.

"I've been busy, too. I'm sorry, but I couldn't wait anymore. I decided that we should go out for dinner tonight." She brushed her palms together.

"Thank you for arranging this. It's a beautiful place," he said, looking around.

"I was thinking we should go shopping soon. I need to buy a new dress for your work Christmas party, and I want you to choose it with me, as usual." She grinned.

"Oh yeah, I almost forgot about it." He checked his calendar on his phone.

"It's on Saturday. Aren't we going?" she asked with darting eyes.

"Yes, we are," he answered.

"How is work?" She ran a hand through her hair.

"It's really busy." He rested his chin on one palm.

"Are you still getting the bad headaches?" Marguerite rested her hand on his.

"Yes." He exhaled.

"I'm sorry, Sébastien. I've just realised that I was so busy that we've forgotten to go for your annual check-up."

"I did see the doctor," he said. He ran a hand through his light brown hair.

"You went by yourself! Why didn't you tell me?" Her forehead puckered.

"You were busy. I didn't want to take you from your students."

"And what did she say? Is everything okay?" she asked.

"Well, she requested many medical tests," he said, while skimming through the menu.

"Then we have to go to the hospital tomorrow to have all the tests done," Marguerite insisted.

"I've done all the tests. I've been to the hospital many times over the last couple of weeks." He ordered two dishes for them and a bottle of wine.

"You have! You never told me. We always do these things together." Disappointment crinkled her eyes.

"This time, I needed to be alone." He lowered his head.

After many years of their marriage, Sébastien had never ceased to admire and respect Marguerite. The fact that she could not bear his children was a misfortune which he had turned into a blessing by uniting them heartily. And while she considered him her only child, he protected her like a father. An electrical engineer, Sébastien sometimes had to travel for work around France and Europe; it was very difficult for Marguerite to handle life without him during his absence.

"So, all the tests were fine, then? You're okay. Right?" She drummed her fingers on the table. Marguerite felt annoyed that he had done all this without her, and probably with someone else.

"They scheduled an operation next week," he said.

"What kind of operation?" she asked.

"Removal of a brain tumour." He rubbed his hands on his thighs.

"Brain tu..." She did not finish the word. Her heart dropped to the floor.

"They'll remove a tumour from my brain." He covered his eyes with his hand.

"What sort of tumour?"

"Cancerous. Then, I'll be on chemotherapy for three months, then radiation."

"When did this happen?" she asked in a strangled voice. Her whole body was shaking.

"Marguerite, please don't make things harder for me than they already are. I've been avoiding this moment. But you have to know. You must be strong." He looked away.

"Do you still love me?" she cried.

"Of course, I do. What are you talking about?" he said, his brows knitting in a frown.

"Never mind," she said, wiping tears on her cheeks. "Tell me, are you in pain now?"

"I am, but it will get worse." He took a sip of his wine.

"I'm so sorry," she groaned, "but after the surgery and the therapy, you'll be fine? Right?"

"Marguerite, I want to be honest with you, but please try to stop crying."

"Tell me that you'll be fine," Marguerite cried.

"Honey, I'm sorry. The doctor says the surgery has a 50% chance."

Speechless, Marguerite sobbed. Sébastien's blue eyes passionately enlarged in silence. Then he continued, "I knew this was going to happen. It's okay, sweetie. Everything will be fine."

"I can't live without you," she said, her head in her hands.

The food came while she was still weeping, and he was holding her affectionately tight in his arms. Still in shock and reluctant to eat, she sat there gazing at every single feature of his face, while he was cutting her steak and feeding her, as he loved to do during their first years together. He was trying his best to calm and reassure her that they would be strong together. She did not cease kissing his hand every time he handed her a bite to eat. After a while, she calmed down, still clinging to his arms.

He then resumed, "We have an appointment at the bank on Monday at 10:00 AM."

"The bank?" Marguerite's eyes enlarged.

"Yes, baby. You have to know all the financial details of our mortgage, monthly expenses, and bill payments." His left arm went around her waist.

"Sébastien, you're not going to leave me alone. You're not. You know I can't live without you," she sobbed again.

"I need you to be strong in order to go through this," he said.

They left the restaurant, their food still on the table half-eaten. Holding hands, they silently looked ahead at their unknown future. They faced the brisk gale, as Marguerite's weary eyes poured heavy tears down her pale cheeks. They walked until they reached Sébastien's car. Driving home, he played one of the many classical music CDs he had in the car. She held his right hand, kissing it constantly, wetting it with her tears. In sorrowful melancholy, she was distressed by the heartbreaking news, yet in priceless gratitude, she was thankful that her assumptions had been wrong.

It was a relief to know that no other woman had stolen his kind heart from her; it was fate that turned her life upside down abruptly. Still, she believed that with their love, they could do miracles and challenge anything. Even death. Nothing on Earth could keep two loving souls apart. Hopeful, she had strong faith that he would survive all this and stay by her side for as long as she would live. She knew he would survive, the operation would succeed, and together they would defeat cancer.

Knowing that his chances to live were 50/50, Sébastien was preparing everything for her to handle life without him. He was worried about her, wondering whether the operation would end his life immediately or only add a few months to it. He drove on the wide Champs Elysées, the lit Eiffel tower getting smaller as he drove farther. Christmas lights, reflecting in the tranquil Seine, brightened up the streets and strengthened the hope in Marguerite's troubled heart. The CD music of Maurice Emmanuel filled the void of silence, offering some comfort to Sébastien's restless mind.

Doubts and Desires

She arrived at her parents' house in the rich, elegant neighbourhood of Rose Bay. It was the last place she wished to be that night, but there was nowhere else for her to go. She parked her small white car in the spacious cul-de-sac in front of a luxurious home, where she had spent all her adolescence.

The overpowering smell of curry, masala, and cardamom came out of the kitchen. It felt suffocating, yet she realised how much she missed her mother and her mouth-watering food. The house was spotless with many bright pictures on the walls. Among them was a family picture of her father sitting down, like King Chandragupta, while she and her mother stood, enclosing him from both sides.

Priya was happy to be early, so she could help her mother. Indrajit was tripping over herself preparing the food, watching the oven in the kitchen, and chopping up vegetables for the salad. She had to make sure that there were many vegetarian choices and enough meat varieties for her husband and others who were not vegan. Priya's father was upstairs relaxing in bed and her grandparents in their room, getting ready for the party. Priya offered to watch the BBQ on the patio, so her mother could finish everything in the kitchen and set the table. They expected the rest of the extended family to arrive in an hour.

In desperate need of fresh air, she escaped the powerful aroma of cumin and coriander in the kitchen and stepped out through the kitchen door onto the patio. It was a nice summer evening — 25°C. Looking down at the spacious backyard, Priya could hardly think of anything but him, wondering what he might be doing right at that moment. Her turquoise and brown paisley dress billowed out around her tiny, short body with the balmy breeze. Her elegant coral necklace and earrings, which she had crafted herself, gleamed around her sad face.

It was a leap year, and that night was the end of it — the New Year's Eve they had planned to spend together. Of all the three hundred and sixty-six days of the year, February 29th was the day they had met for the first time. The anniversary of that dear memory would not recur but once every fourth year. At first she had considered that exceptionally unique. This was the beginning of their relationship, which had begun fast and strong, remaining intense and ambivalent.

Emmanuel lay down on the couch in a small apartment shared with his currently out-of-town roommate, trying to convince himself that he was sleeping. His phone had not stopped ringing. His mother had called and left a message asking him to come over and spend New Year's Eve with them if he was home alone. A couple of his friends had also left messages, wondering if he had plans that night, and giving him other suggestions if he did not. Hearing his phone ringing on the kitchen counter, he lacked the motivation to get up and see who was calling.

Priya stood on the deck to watch the BBQ. Looking at the glaze of the coal burning under the meat, she remembered the many situations when he had caused her embarrassment and discomfort. She recalled the last time they had seen each other a week earlier. They were shopping at the Westfield Paramatta Mall when she met a friend of hers. She innocently stopped to say hello and introduced him to Emmanuel. Suddenly, the latter excused himself and walked away. Priya got troubled. "There we go again," she murmured.

She could not guess what she did to make him angry. She continued talking to her friend, her eyes fixed on Emmanuel until he disappeared completely. Saying goodbye, she went after Emmanuel, walking fast in the crowded mall. She finally found him sitting on a bench talking to a woman. Priya had no idea who she was. Emmanuel was laughing with her and opening a new subject every time she tried to end the conversation and leave. The woman eventually left. Priya approached to sit by his side, while he was reading some brochures, ignoring her.

"What's wrong?" Priya asked.

"I don't know," he bluntly answered.

"Why did you leave?" she asked.

"You were talking to your friend," he answered, looking down at the brochures.

"Mike was my classmate at school." She pressed a hand to her throat.

"Did I ask you?" he yelled, slamming his fists on the bench.

"Alright, let's go and cook dinner at my place," Priya suggested.

"Cook? Do you think you know how to cook?" He laughed.

"What's wrong with you?"

"Nothing, I said. I'm fine," he yelled once more.

"Fine. Let's go then," she said.

"No, I'm not coming. I'm going home." He left her sitting on the bench by herself, without explaining what the problem was.

She had not heard from him since. She decided not to call this time. They were supposed to be together now celebrating New Year's Eve. He did not care to ask her to come over as they had planned. It was becoming too hard for Priya. She could not tolerate it anymore knowing that this relationship was toxic and harmful to her self-esteem and well-being.

He had made her suffer, and Priya decided to help herself get over him by remembering everything he had done. His jealousy became too possessive. His un-controlled anger troubled her inner peace. She recalled every time she felt tongue-tied when he yelled at her to answer him fast. The tone of his voice when he asked her an unexpected question made her brain freeze up. His response to her simple mistakes irritated her. She often felt too intimidated to suggest an idea to him because she feared his reactions. She hated when he put her down and made fun of her opinions and views. She felt so stupid after his daunting remarks and sarcastic comments attacked her talents and abilities.

Emmanuel rose at last and went to check his phone, to find tens of missed calls and messages from many people except her. He put the phone on the table, turning the ringer off. He walked to his bedroom and looked at the empty bed. He and Priya were supposed to be there now — making love. He organised some files and books on the desk. On the crowded bookshelves, his PhD degree certificate was almost falling among big math textbooks. He picked it up, looked at it for a minute. He read every word on it and put it back on the desk. He turned the air conditioner off and opened the window. A nice breeze billowed in. Then he went and took a cool shower.

The shower soothed his body, but his mind was still all over the place. He went to the living room, grabbed the bottle of scotch, sat on the couch, and turned on the TV. Half an hour passed as he mindlessly flipped through channels, trying to find anything interesting to captivate his mind, until he found an action movie that was just starting.

The lamb and chicken Priya was grilling were perfectly done, so she turned the BBQ off and came back into the kitchen, which was already spotlessly clean. Her mom went to take a quick shower and dress, while Priya arranged her jewellery sets to display on the corner table of the living room, with the hope that her relatives would be interested in buying some.

Eighteen years earlier, when Priya was ten, her parents had moved to Sydney, Australia to make a better life for their one and only daughter. Rich and well-educated, her father had managed to build a prestigious career as a veterinarian and provided a decent life for his family. Her mother had never worked outside the home, having generously dedicated her life to her husband, her daughter, and her parents-in-law. Growing up, Priya suffered confusing cultural conflicts through her teenage years.

The doorbell rang, and she was there to greet the visitors — all the extended family on both her parents' side. As the guests came in, Priya received chocolates — one box after another. Her favourite was the caramel chocolate with hazelnut, which she ate while greeting her relatives.

She was relieved when Jea arrived. She was the only person with whom Priya could talk freely; they had been very close as teenagers. Priya hugged her and said, "Jea, so good to see you." They talked, catching up on their news. "How is Charita?" Priya asked.

"She's getting married in April. She should be here soon with Neerav." Jea looked around.

"How are they getting along? Do you think she's happy?" Priya asked, narrow-eyed.

"She's very happy and excited, actually," Jea answered, surprised by Priya's question.

"I can't imagine myself with an Indian man." Priya rubbed her forehead.

"I don't feel that way." Jea arched a sly brow.

"You didn't have your grandparents living with you." Priya turned her face away and continued, "I didn't like seeing my mother serving them every meal and then cleaning up after them. My father never offered to help."

"My parents are different. They have a balanced marriage as far as I can see. They share responsibilities and have good communication." Jea picked a piece of chocolate from the opened box by the half wall near the entrance.

"I always had a feeling that Mom stayed with Dad out of fear rather than love." Priya played with her phone.

"This may only be your perception, Priya. To me, Auntie Indrajit seems content and satisfied," Jea disagreed.

"If she's satisfied, that's only because she never had the courage to leave. I always felt alienated by that culture," said Priya, running her hand through her long hair.

"But look at my mother. She and Auntie are sisters, raised in the same house by the same parents, yet they're very different. Mom is a successful business woman who established a career. So, don't blame it on the culture, please," Jea argued, her arms crossed.

"Your father is open-minded and modern. Plus, you were born and raised here. You didn't have to switch between two different societies. My experience was different. When I was twenty, I left and found a place to live on my own. Dad didn't talk to me for two years." Priya rolled her eyes.

"I'm glad things are better now. It's been seven years. How is your jewellery-making going?" Jea asked.

"Come have a look. I brought some sets with me to show you," said Priya.

Priya, smart and talented, lacked the most important thing of all — self-confidence. She always doubted herself and her abilities. Everybody around her told her she was skillfully gifted at designing and crafting jewellery, but she hardly believed in her potential. She barely managed to silence her own self-doubts, let alone Emmanuel's dispiriting opinions and discouraging words. Yet she always held on to her dream to become a jewellery designer.

The table was set, and dinner was served. The meal was delicious. Priya tried every dish on the table and had seconds of the butter chicken that she never ate away from that house. After dinner, she helped with cleaning up and serving desserts. Again, she could not resist the countless pies, cakes, and sweets that everybody brought in. It was a night full of food, family memories, jokes, songs, dancing, and chocolate until midnight. All this helped to temporarily take her mind away from Emmanuel.

When the clock struck twelve, Emmanuel was falling asleep on the couch. The TV was still on and loud. The empty whisky bottle lay on the floor.

All the visitors left right after midnight. The house was quiet again, but messy. Her father and grandparents went to their rooms, but Priya stayed to help Indrajit clean everything so the house would look decently organised the next morning. Thirty minutes later, she took two plastic bags full of leftovers that her mother had packed, kissed her as she wished her a Happy New Year, and off she drove.

Priya, in her car, and Emmanuel, in a dream, both viewed their intimate moments. In bed, they were wildly in sync. The harmony between their bodies was rare. He could not find similar delight with another woman, nor did she feel comparable enjoyment with another man. They could spend hours making love without getting bored or tired. He never got tired of kissing every inch of her spicy skin, and she never got bored of feeling his strong hands all over her juicy body. When their flaming bodies united, the bedroom turned into a volcano of suppressed emotions, erupting in the middle of a vast, raging ocean.

Although her brain knew that their relationship was not meant to last, and her soul was never comfortable around him, her body was pulling her toward his like the negative edge of a magnet.

She was not surprised that she hardly felt sleepy after all the caffeine and sugar. It was a moonless night with clear sky. She went to the bathroom to take a cool shower. Still not feeling sleepy, she played some Indian songs, which reminded her of her childhood when she was still in India. The energetic music caused her slim arms to softly move up and down, her sexy legs to take rhythmic steps back and forth, and her hips and waist to shake delicately left and right. She danced insanely. Her soft long black hair and her loose colourful nightgown danced in the air along with her body. Her big brown eyes brightly shone under her thick eyebrows and wide russet forehead. Her full, sweet lips sang along with the lyrics. She was a lively illustration of goddess Lakshmi. Not realising how much time had passed, she crashed on her bed as breezes blew through the wide open window.

Early next morning, Emmanuel woke to the sound of birds in the bushes around the building where he lived. The streets were placid; everyone was sleeping after the long night. He always awakened too early. He barely slept in the first place, and in the midst of his sleep, his brain was always awake, with one of his eyes slightly open. He stayed still for a short while, thinking of Priya. Feelings of guilt hit his heart, and thoughts of loss invaded his head. Looking around, he realised that he was still on the couch and the TV was on; it was time for the national news. Dragging his tall body, he rose with difficulty, walked to the table and grabbed his phone.

He went through all the missed calls and the voice and text messages, only to find none from her. Had he lost her forever? He could hardly believe it. *Why didn't she call this time?* he wondered. She had such a big heart that could always find excuses for him.

He missed her terribly, but he did not know what to do. He could not call her. He only hoped she would call. He desperately fancied her showing up on his doorstep. His heart ached, and his brain was paralysed. He picked a name from the contact list on his phone, hit the message button, and typed, "Hey Rebecca, Happy New Year. Do you want to meet up for coffee?" After clicking on the send arrow, he looked at the clock — it was 5:00 AM. "Damn it, of course she's sleeping."

Now there was no way he could go back to sleep, even though he tried. He made coffee, watched the news, but failed to get Priya out of his head. If it was possible to do that any other time, it was impossible that day. It was a holiday. Everything was closed. Everyone was sleeping.

Nobody was there to talk to, nowhere to go, nothing to do. He was going insane, every tick of the clock stoning the vain temple of his body.

Five hours later, which seemed like five decades, he received a text message from Rebecca, "Hello, Emmanuel, Happy New Year. I'd love to go for coffee, but where? All the coffee shops are closed today."

Rebecca was one of the very few friends Emmanuel succeeded in keeping; he felt more comfortable talking to her than to anyone else. She was patient with him, even when he was irritated. She knew how to calm him down, listen to what he wanted to say, and say what he needed to hear. He called Rebecca and said Happy New Year.

"What did you do last night?" Rebecca asked.

"Nothing," he answered.

"How is it going with Priya?" she asked.

"We're not talking."

"Again!" Rebecca gasped.

Having known him since their adolescence, Rebecca knew that Emmanuel hurt others because he was hurting, and although he deserved the least love, he needed it the most. Ironically, Rebecca used to have a crush on Emmanuel years earlier, but when he started seeing other girls, she was satisfied with staying his close friend. Still, talking about another girl was painful, especially since she had broken up with her boyfriend two weeks earlier.

"The last time I saw her was a week ago. Had she called, I would've apologised," he said.

"She's had enough, Emmanuel. She can't be the one to run after you every time you leave her. This time, you should've called her. Especially that it was New Year's Eve."

"I can't call her. I said very hurtful words to her last time. I said to her that she was a failure, and I called her stupid." Emmanuel rubbed his shoulder.

"Why?" Rebecca asked, irritated.

"I don't know. Her slow responses drive me insane. I get very impatient when she takes forever to think or decide. I'm a fast-paced person. My life is go, go, go. She's very hesitant and doubtful. She doesn't even get my jokes or sarcasm. She's too sensitive." He gripped the arm of the chair.

"Do you love her or not?" Rebecca asked.

"I miss her touch. I love her body. I want her. She's awesome," said Emmanuel, hand fondling his private parts.

"She's not only a body, Emmanuel. She's a person. She has feelings."

"I know. I hurt her feelings. Many times. I feel terrible now. She's kind and caring. She's forgiving. She's a sweetheart. She knows how to make me happy." He rubbed his chin.

"Then call her and say you're sorry," Rebecca suggested.

"I can't call her. I can't handle rejection. It's too late now. I wish I'd called last night. If she'd cared, she would've called. I think that's it for our relationship."

Emmanuel was not truly as self-confident as he appeared to those around him; deep inside, he felt terrifyingly insecure. He attempted to gain this fake self-confidence by demoralising everybody he knew, and of course, Priya was his first prey. The voice of his mother rang in his ears every now and then, talking to him in Spanish when he was still in elementary school: *You have to be the best in class!* And if another student got better marks than he, she would rebuke him in a harsh way. She was a tough mother, and she became tougher after his father had left them and disappeared when Emmanuel was a teenager — the oldest of his three siblings.

Aware that he was handsome and attractive to women, Emmanuel spent hours in the gym building muscles to look younger, more seductive. His academic success was not enough to make him feel adequately secure, to help others up, instead of putting them down and proving that he was better. As smart as he was in school, he lacked emotional intelligence in human relations. And despite his high education, he failed to keep a decent job. He ran a small business — Emmanuel Fernandez for Life Coaching — bearing his name, the two most important words for him, which barely made enough money to survive.

Priya slowly opened her eyes and looked at the clock; the hour hand pointed ten, and the minute hand six. The rays of the sun penetrated the dullness of her disorganised bedroom, as the phone ringtone disturbed the silence. She looked at her phone to see who it was. "Oh Melanie!" she tearfully voiced her relief that finally she could talk to someone and let all her emotions out. She had imprisoned her feelings inside for so long that it was becoming achingly unbearable.

She swiftly hit the answer button and said, "Melanie, I miss you so much."

Melanie replied in her cheerful and positive voice, "Hi Priya, Happy New Year."

"I need to talk to you now more than ever," Priya replied. Melanie suggested that Priya go to her house for a coffee and a quick late breakfast or an early lunch.

Priya got up quickly, and was ready in half an hour, during which Melanie managed to prepare a simple meal for them to share after coffee. Priya arrived at her small, cozy house by the Paramatta River. Melanie hugged her at the door; Priya was silently weeping. She did not care to hide her tears. By then, she needed nothing in the world but to let them flow. She had been strong for so long.

Melanie let Priya in, and they had coffee. "I love the smell of coffee," Priya said, trying to smile with her lips but unable to make her tired eyes copy them. "I miss the days when we worked together, when you used to make coffee every morning in the office."

They sat down chatting and catching up on their news until his name came up when Melanie asked, "What did you do last night for New Year's Eve?"

"I spent it at my parents'. They had a big party for the whole family. It was nice," Priya replied.

"Is Emmanuel out of town?" Melanie asked.

"No. He's here, but we haven't been talking since last week."

"Why am I not surprised?" Melanie said.

"He didn't even call last night. We were planning to spend the night together because his roommate is out of town." Priya looked at something in the air between them that Melanie could not spot.

"He'll never call. He's expecting you to call," said Melanie, rolling her eyes.

"This time I really can't call him. I've had enough of this. I was strong the whole week until this morning. Now I miss him again." Frustration crinkled Priya's eyes.

"He's not the right person for you. His pride is a barrier standing between you and him. His ego is huge, taking such a big space in his head that there's no room for reason. He's a narcissist." Melanie looked away.

"I know we're not for each other," Priya said.

"Do you really? I've heard you say that before."

"The problem is, I don't know how to get over him. My life is not the same when he's not in it." Priya buried her hands in her hair.

"He hurts your feelings and discourages you," Melanie reminded her.

"You're right. But he also makes me laugh. He cares for me. I miss his constant messages and calls. My phone doesn't ring now," said Priya, wrapping her arms around herself.

"You're just used to his presence in your life. It's going to take some time until you get used to his absence."

"I know he won't call me. He's too proud and stubborn." Priya punched the cushion.

"What if he calls? What will you do?" Melanie asked.

"He won't call. I'm sure he's with another girl now," Priya's lip quivered. "Anyway, I feel better now that I talked with you about it. I needed to cry. That helped a lot. It's a relief. I'll be fine." Priya drew in a long breath.

Priya had a good amount of jewellery sets in her car from the previous night, so she went out to bring some in for Melanie. They were uniquely designed and skillfully crafted. Priya laid her bracelets, necklaces, and earrings on the coffee table in an artistic way; the stones looked like flowers of all colours and shapes. Priya used real onyx stones to make her jewellery sets, so they were more expensive than people expected, but Melanie knew that and insisted on buying an antique burgundy set from her.

Seeing and talking to Melanie, and the fact that she had bought that set from her improved Priya's mood immensely. Melanie was not worried about Priya any longer; she knew Priya was one of two extremes — submissive or rebellious — she either stayed silent and helpless, or rebelled and fled.

Priya said goodbye and left. She felt invigorated, ready to go home and work on her jewellery. Knowing it would be painful, she still determined not to think about Emmanuel again.

Emmanuel went out for a walk by himself. The streets were deserted and boring. He came home to the empty apartment. All memories started to jumble in his head again, and the pain of missing Priya ached in his heart. He grabbed his phone to check but found nothing from her. That was when he started to go through their text messages, until his finger hit the call button by mistake. He panicked. Swiftly, he wanted to hit the end-call button. But in a moment he thought, *nothing is a mistake in this world. I'll talk to her.*

Love, Learn and Laugh

It was Friday, one week before Easter, when she decided to go alone on a trip to visit the city she had always wanted to see. She lay on the couch in her small apartment. Four empty water bottles were on the coffee table. The TV was on. With her phone in her hand, she went through all the text messages she had received from him during the last six months.

She was exhausted from wandering for hours on Whyte Ave. She walked aimlessly, trying to hide herself among the crowd and the falling snowflakes. She was too shocked to comprehend what had just happened. It was a dreadful night — the night James broke up with Marissa after an extraordinary love story that had lasted only a few months.

In tearless disbelief, she was staring at the background picture of her phone — a photo of them together by the frozen Saskatchewan River in downtown Edmonton, when he was last in town. She remembered all the memories she had shared with James, how he suddenly erupted in her still life and then abruptly disappeared. Hating to see herself in this helpless state of mind, she got up, went straight to her laptop, and started to search for a reasonably-priced flight ticket.

After searching and comparing prices, she finally made her choice and booked her flight to Seattle, departing the following day in the early afternoon. By that time, it was already 1:00 AM. She went and opened the window; the cold breeze was fresh and kind to her fair skin and flew gently through her wavy chestnut hair. It had finally stopped snowing; a glittering thick white carpet covered the ground. The fluffy snowflakes covered every inch of the branches, and the trees looked like ladies in shimmering wedding dresses. Although the scene was beautiful, it was somewhat frustrating. *Will Spring ever come?* she thought. She took a deep breath, trying to snap out of that agonising pain and looking up to the sky she saw the full moon.

She gloomily chuckled, "I knew it. It's the full moon! That explains everything." She could hold her tears no more. Closing the window, she bitterly cried, recalling every moment they spent together, every word he said to her, and every touch.

When they met that evening, he was depressed and lost in thought. He was someone else — a merciless person. He flew from Victoria to Edmonton to break up with her face to face. Cruelly, he told her he could not continue with their relationship, that he was not ready for a commitment and could not endure the challenges. Their relationship was more complicated than he could handle, and he could not promise her anything.

The next morning, she woke up to the sound of the radio beside her bed; it was 7:00 AM. She had hardly slept two complete hours, but she had to get up and pack. Her flight was only a few hours away. She rushed out of bed, showered, dressed and had her coffee in about forty-five minutes; she was ready. Her attractive silhouette looked good in her blue sweater and tight dark jeans, but her hazel eyes seemed fatigued and absent. She packed her small suitcase. She was only going to stay there for three days over the weekend, plus an extra day she managed to take off.

She left, taking the bus to the airport, and arrived very early for her flight. She checked in, walked to the gate, and sat down, waiting for boarding time which was an hour away. She took out a book she had bought two weeks earlier but had not yet read. Looking at the pages, she could not see the words; all she could see was a flashback of her life story.

Lost in empty space, she suddenly heard the flight attendant calling her name: *Ms. Marissa Lardeau, Ms. Marissa Lardeau.* Embarrassed, she answered, "Yes." She could not believe she had lost track of time and that the plane was waiting for her. She collected her belongings, ran to the gate, and showing her passport and boarding pass, quickly stepped onto the plane.

She looked for her seat number and was relieved when she found the seat next to her empty. She wanted to be alone, even during the plane ride. A few seconds after she settled in her seat and made herself comfortable, a good-looking middle-aged man came and sat beside her. *Apparently, I'm not going to enjoy my own company for the next two hours,* she thought.

As soon as the plane took off, the gentleman kindly smiled at her and said, "Hello." Reluctantly, she said, "Hi," and turned her head the other way, looking through the tight window. The view of the rays of the sun intermingling with the clouds offered a perfect dimension for her to vanish into.

George Whitmore, a professor of Geography, was on his way to Seattle for a one-day work trip. Curious by nature, he wanted to know more about the book that Marissa was pretending to read and to chat with her, passing time until they reached their destination.

He started by asking, "So, are you going to Seattle for work or vacation?"

"Mini vacation," she answered.

"Do you have family there?" he asked.

"No," she said.

"Are you from Edmonton?" She shook her head.

"Where are you from?" he asked.

"Montreal," she answered.

"Were you born in Montreal?" he asked.

"No," she said.

"Where were you born?" he wondered.

"Spain. My mother came to Canada when I was five," she said, looking away — but he did not stop.

"Oh, so you're actually Spanish."

She nodded, "My mother is Spanish, and my father is French."

"I moved to Alberta ten years ago," he said. "I like it here; it's beautiful, especially in the summertime."

George had left England for a prestigious job offer to teach at the University of Alberta. Full of youth and enthusiasm, his outgoing personality suited his profession. He enjoyed talking to his students about almost every subject in life, not just Geography. He had just celebrated his fiftieth birthday a week earlier with his two daughters, who had come all the way from England to share that special day with him. He had been very happy to see them after such a long time.

He continued and asked, "What made you move to Edmonton, then?"

"Work," she said.

"What do you do for a living?"

"I'm a French Teacher." She inspected her fingernail.

By that time, Marissa seriously started to feel an uncomfortable pressure. She excused herself to go to the washroom and left the book face down on her seat. Curious to know who the author was, George peeked at the book to read the book pitch on the back cover. Since it took her quite a while, he went on to read the first page. When he smelled the delightful scent of Marissa's perfume invading his nostrils, he put the book back on her seat and stood up to let her in. Quietly Marissa slid into her seat, thinking it was not such a bad idea to chat with that intriguing fellow who did not want to stop talking. He wanted to apologise for taking her book, so he said, "Sorry, I was just curious to check the book you're reading."

"No problem," she said.

"Love, Learn, and Laugh! A very catchy title! Is it an inspiring novel?" he asked.

"I don't know," she stammered.

"You don't know?" he said, puzzled.

"I mean, I haven't started reading it. I just read the preface," she said.

"I have a feeling it's very thought-provoking, even though I don't know the author."

"I've seen her speak at a conference for international writers in New York. This is her first published book."

"International writers! Where is she from?" he asked

"She lives in the States, but she's originally from Colombia."

"So, this is a translated text then," he assumed.

"No. This is the original text. She writes in English," she said.

"Interesting!" He scratched his nose.

Marissa felt tired and sleepy; she had hardly rested the previous night. Hearing her stomach growl, she remembered that she had not eaten anything since lunch on the previous day, and she started to feel hungry too. The aroma of coffee woke her up when the flight attendants passed by with the drinks and food carts. Marissa asked for coffee and purchased a sandwich. She was emotionally drained and physically exhausted. George asked for tea and drank it while flipping the pages of the *Globe and Mail.* In an attempt to revive the conversation, he thought of talking about the book one more time.

"Love. It is good to love. Isn't it? How do you define love?" he asked.

"It's something that doesn't exist," she answered, looking away.

"Oh! This is so unfair. You're too young to come to such a shocking conclusion," George said, arms crossed.

"I'm not young; I am thirty-five."

"Thirty-five, and you think you're not young." George laughed and continued, "Yes, you are. Why do you say love doesn't exist?"

"The reality is, we blindly fall in love with people we know nothing about, and then we gradually start falling out of love with them the moment we get to know them better," she said, wrapping her arms around herself.

"You're talking exclusively about love between a man and a woman. Aren't you?" George commented, stroking his chin.

"There's no love between a man and a woman; it's just desire. For men, it is a fiery passion that starts in a second and ends in another second, living for a very short time in between. And sometimes it is also an adventure that doesn't last longer than a few months." She played with her cellphone.

"And for women?" George asked.

"For women, it is the need to feel secure, appreciated, and satisfied. And nine times out of ten, women don't feel secure, appreciated, or satisfied in relationships."

"I can tell you're talking from a bad experience, but that doesn't mean every relationship you'll have will be the same. The past has passed. *Tourne la page!*"

"In every story, the beginning will always be beautiful, but it won't last; it will remain 'a beginning' forever."

Marissa heard her mother's gentle voice repeating, "Happy endings are stories that haven't ended yet." Her mother was her heroine; she had raised her after having moved from Europe to Quebec as a single mother, facing all the challenges and overcoming every obstacle alone.

"There are no endings," he said, "but rather, a series of new beginnings. Nothing lasts forever, yet everything is the same. It's the life cycle. Do you have children?"

"No, I don't," she said.

It was getting too dismal for Marissa. She turned her head the other way and could not help letting tears slip down her pale cheeks. All her friends were in relationships and had children of their own, and there she was alone and childless. It was tough for her to find a reason to live for. She had no purpose in life. She thought of James again. She missed him terribly. Her heart was aching; she was tormented by the thought of not having him in her life any longer.

They both knew from the very beginning that their relationship was complicated, and that there were some obstacles to overcome. Yet he had always told her that he knew she was the right woman for him, and that he felt strong and safe with her. He called her "the woman of my dreams". He said she was different from all the women he had met before. He said he was sure their roads had crossed for a reason, and that she had appeared in his life at the perfect moment.

And she believed him. She believed him because she wanted to believe him. She was in desperate need of someone to care for her, and he cared. He cared, as nobody else did. He was thoughtful and compassionate. He gave her all his attention and time. How could he change suddenly after such a short time? And why? The circumstances were the same from day one. Nothing had changed.

Marissa then turned to George and continued, "Well, to have children, I need to find their father first."

"You will," he said.

"I've stopped looking."

"He'll find you."

"I'm not waiting anymore." She shrugged.

"Don't wait! Let him find you while you're busy doing something else."

"By that time, I'll be too old to have children."

"No, you won't. Plus, having children is not the only purpose in life. Having your own children and finding yourself are two unrelated issues."

"My life is empty and meaningless." She sighed.

Marissa had known that James would eventually leave her, yet she had never expected the day to come so soon. Part of her understood why he had come to that conclusion and why he was too tired to continue the long journey with her. She could not blame him for not loving her sincerely enough to face the challenges. But she believed in their love; she felt stronger with him. She was ready to move to another province to be closer to him. But after six months he had realised that he would not be able to handle a long-distance relationship, not even temporarily.

"Love doesn't necessarily have to be for a person," George continued; "it can be for something. Your passion!

119

Which probably brings us to the next word in the title of your book: Learn."

"Learn what?" Marissa asked, forehead puckered.

"What is your gift?" he asked, his hands clasped tight in front of his chest.

"I don't have a gift," she said.

"Everybody has a gift. You just need to find out what it is. By learning new skills, you'll find out: playing a musical instrument, for example, painting, writing, fashion designing, learning a new language. Anything!"

"I don't think I am interested in any of this." She closed the book and put it in her purse.

"What are you good at doing?"

"My friends say I am a good listener; they always like to come and talk to me when they're in trouble. I regret not getting a degree in psychology. I would have enjoyed being a psychologist. It's too late now, anyway." Marissa shrugged.

"You still can get a second degree in psychology if you really want to, but if you can't make it a profession, make it a devotion. Talk and listen to people in distress; you can change lives by just doing that. Contact associations where you can volunteer."

"I'll think about it."

"To live is to learn. Life has no worth if we don't learn something new every day. Being a professor makes me a learner, too. I teach my students, and I learn from them."

"No matter how much we learn," she argued, "certain things in life will always remain mysteries." She rested her chin in her palm.

"You're right," he agreed, "but that doesn't mean we should stop asking questions or searching for answers."

"Life is hilariously heartbreaking. What someone is dreaming of and hoping for is the same thing that someone else is regretting or considering a mistake to fix," she said, as she ran her left hand through her hair.

"Life is hilariously heartbreaking, but I'd rather laugh at it than let it make me cry. Life is a joke. Even if you don't get it, just laugh!" he tittered.

"If it is a joke, it is not even funny," she said, lips curled.

"But remember, behind every joke, there's some truth. I hope you'll enjoy your book. Don't forget to love, learn, and laugh! That's exactly how your soul stays young forever," he said, smiling with his eyes and mouth.

Before they knew it, the plane was already landing at the Seattle International Airport. After they got off the plane and received their luggage, they said goodbye, and each of them went in a different direction. George took a cab to the hotel where the conference would take place, while Marissa walked to the bus stop.

She inhaled a lovely scent that was familiar; she looked around and found the Seattle Airport Florist, where they had pots of basil out on the sidewalk in the sun. That was the second time she remembered her mother that day; her mother had always kept a basil plant in a pot in their kitchen. Marissa decided that her next trip would have to be to Montreal to see her. She got on the bus to the hotel, where she would be staying for the next two nights. The bus ride was long, but she enjoyed it greatly and was thrilled to view the streets of Seattle.

The bus passed by the Duwamish River she had read about. The white sailboats in the river, moved by the soft wind, gently energised the water, which had been abandoned during many weeks of cold long nights. The warm breeze carried the good news to the birds; they could leave their nests to sing and dance with the wind. After having been away for all the months of winter, they came home to the sky that belonged to them. The smell of rain announced the rebirth of the bare branches of the trees and bushes. The sun was warm and tender, and the tall trees were budding, kindly providing some shade for people walking under them.

She saw the famous Pike Place Fish Market. Discovering where it was, she decided to go visit it the following day and have a fresh seafood meal for lunch. She was already feeling better; thinking of James was not hurting as badly as before. *Oh well. If he can't value my love or go through some temporary difficulties, then too bad*, she said to herself.

Marissa looked at her book and wondered what it was about. She was eager to read it over the following three days and compare the real content with her interesting conversation with that unusual man. She wondered if one day they would run across each other in Edmonton, or maybe she could even look him up. Spontaneously, she grabbed her phone to google his name, when all of a sudden she burst into loud laughter. She did not know what his name was. Marissa and George had talked for almost two hours but hadn't introduced themselves.

Home and Heart

Her eyelids reluctantly moved upward and downward as the alarm went off. It was six o'clock. As she yawned, she blinked nervously when she remembered. After work she was going on a date that she had been deliberately postponing for several weeks, but could not delay any longer. He had called her the day before and insisted that they should meet.

One of her friends had connected her with someone who, she thought, would make a good partner for Shiva, but the latter was not sure about that. Since she had heard his name, she had been hesitant to welcome the opportunity. His identity took her on a trip down memory lane, full of wistful moments of bright sunrises and foggy ones of dark storms.

She showered and dried her hair. She put on the floral basil and peach outfit, her gold chain with a pendant of Anahita, and the amethyst jewellery set. She looked at the pendant in the mirror and laughed; she always wished her name was 'Anahita'.

Thankful it was Friday, she arrived at work and received many compliments from her colleagues about how good she looked. It was going to be a busy day, although work was usually slower in July. She finished her morning appointments and went for lunch instead of going for her daily walk to San Francisco Bay.

In the lunchroom, Crystal, also a psychologist at UCSF Women's Health Centre, joined her. They talked about work while eating. "The hardest thing about our job is the challenge to keep an unbiased attitude and try to understand both sides of an argument," Shiva said, as she told Crystal about a mysterious client of hers.

"And the best thing about our job is knowing that what most of them have gone through makes us feel thankful for the life we've had," Crystal added.

"You're right. We can't complain. I'll be alright once I find an apartment to move to. The landlord has decided not to renew the rent and move in instead," said Shiva, her curly eyelashes surrounded her worried brown eyes.

"You'll be even happier when you find a soulmate." Crystal tittered.

"A home is more important." Shiva shook her head. She had been accustomed to living alone.

"Who knows, maybe you'll find both at the same time. Usually these things happen when you least expect, where you least expect." Crystal winked.

"I had a strange dream last night. I just remembered now." Shiva slapped her forehead. "I was in a house that I'd never seen before."

"It's a new life waiting for you." Crystal became excited.

"It was an older, yet elegant three-storey house. There were large windows in all the rooms, overlooking the bay." Shiva grinned.

"Maybe that will be your new house," Crystal teased her. "Yeah right," Shiva jested, "I can barely afford to rent a two-bedroom apartment. The rent has gone up in just the last few months. It's crazy."

The day went by quickly; it was busier than usual because of the Mental Health Awareness week at the hospital.

Shiva was not certain how she felt about her date; she experienced nostalgic yearning mingled with burdened aching. She wanted to go anyway, yet she did not want to have high hopes dashed. She left work and went to the Blue Mermaid House which she had suggested to him the previous evening on the phone. She arrived a bit early, as the restaurant was a very short drive from where she worked. She was seated at a table for two on the terrace, facing San Francisco Bay.

A few minutes later, Dr. Salehi arrived. He spotted her in no time and went confidently to greet her, then seated himself after taking his blazer off. They exchanged some glances while talking about how the day went. They both knew the basic personal information about each other. Hamed was a successful psychiatrist who earned a reputation among his patients for his devotion to his work and dedication to them.

They had seen each other's photos, but it was still different to see each other in person. Shiva found Hamed handsome. It was hard to believe that he was retiring in three years. And he thought she was energetic and beautiful; she barely looked one day older than forty. The way Hamed talked reminded Shiva of her father. His laughter took her decades back. She scented the fragrance of carnations in the garden of their house, and saw herself playing with her brother and cousins, when they were innocent and free. Her taste buds savoured her grandmother's sweet *samanu*. Hamed was comforted to feel at home.

They were greeted by their host for the evening. They both ordered their meals after they were given some time to read the menu. Before the waitress left the table, Shiva asked her for separate bills. Hamed heard this, but it was too late for him to say otherwise. When Shiva sensed his hidden discomfort, she learned the first thing about his personality — traditional, unlike her. She managed to keep an agreeable smile on her face all the time.

In a few seconds, he decided to express how he felt. "Why did you ask for separate bills? I'm willing to pay the whole bill. It's my pleasure," he gently said.

"Thank you. It's very kind of you, but its okay," Shiva said.

"Why?" Hamed asked, perplexed.

"Why do you feel you have to pay?" Shiva wondered.

"Well, it's not that I have to, but I'd love to," he said.

"Why?" Shiva asked again.

"I am a man. A Muslim man." He chuckled.

"Muslim!" Shiva said, eyebrows raised. "The best memory I have of Islam is Khadija, the first wife of Muhammad. Didn't she propose to him and share with him all her wealth?"

"Yeah, you're right." He scratched his nose.

"Why do you think men have to pay for women then? Where did that come from?" She crossed her legs and tossed her wavy black hair over her straight shoulders.

"I invited you to dinner." He leaned forward.

"No, you didn't. We both agreed to meet up for dinner." She reclined in her seat.

"The Quran says, 'Men are in charge of women'." He smiled and asked, "Have you read the Quran?"

Traditional and religious, Shiva silently murmured, and continued, "Oh yes, I've read the Quran. I came from a Muslim family in Iran."

Shiva had left Iran twenty-nine years earlier and had now lived half of her life in the USA. Her lifestyle and mentality were more American, yet her face was authentic Persian. Dr. Salehi, on the other hand, had left Tehran twenty years earlier, but Iran had never left him. He had been living in San Francisco for all these years with the mentality and lifestyle of a typical Iranian person.

"But I'm not practising Islam," Shiva quickly clarified, as she sipped some cool water. Her grip on the edge of the table tightened.

"I see. May I ask why?" Hamed softly asked.

"Well, I don't practise any religion. I don't think it's a good idea." Shiva giggled. "More wars have started in the name of religion than for any other reason." She twisted her ring.

"Both World Wars I and II that caused the largest destruction in human history had nothing to do with religion. They were fighting over ethnicities and lands," Hamed reasoned, placing the tips of his fingers together.

"Maybe, but I still don't like the concept of an authority controlling people's lives," Shiva said, her lips pressed.

"I don't look at it as a controlling authority," Hamed disagreed, "I'm a simple Muslim. To me, Islam is to live with love in peace." His silver hair shone in the sun rays.

"Do you think the Islamic State that slaughters people and burn them alive represents love and peace?" She gave a sarcastic smile.

"The Islamic State is not Islam." He laughed. "They're an evil gang." Hamed said, stroking his chin.

"Why do they call themselves the Islamic State then?" Shiva tapped her fingers and continued, "And it's not just them," Shiva went on, "the Islamic governments in the Middle East arrest and kill thousands of youths, whip people, and cut their legs and arms in public." She turned her face away.

"Well, they too only want authority and power. They are no different from the corrupt church of the Middle

Ages," Hamed replied with a smile.

"That's why Islam is in tremendous danger," she said; "it'll never be saved unless enlightened Muslims like you protect their own religion." Shiva folded her arms.

"I agree, but realistically speaking, we can only do so much. Unfortunately, those who have the power to change don't want to change anything. But the truth is many Muslim people desire nothing but to live in peace." He leaned back in his chair.

"That's true, but not enough. I think it's their responsibility to protect Islam. Otherwise, they shouldn't call themselves Muslims." Shiva sipped some more cold water as she continued, "I know the majority of Muslims aren't fanatic, but about 20% of them are. Do you know how many that percentage makes? Do the math!" Shiva's breath quickened.

Their conversation took a path that carried to Shiva troublesome memories. She could not hide her discomfort with fake smiles any longer. She could not unsee the image of her brother's face, flickering in front of her eyes. She excused herself to go wash her hands before eating. She went to the restroom and turned on the cold water tap and spent a few minutes washing her hands. Her eyes were lost in the reflection of the water, running down the white sink.

She smelt the rotten walls of the prison. She heard the sound of shootings on the streets of Tehran. She saw the heartbroken faces of mothers who lost their children, and the innocent tears of children who lost their parents. Everything about Hamed reminded her of Iran, the good days and the bad ones. *I knew this was going to happen*, she regretted. She breathed deeply in and out, looking out through a large window beside the restroom until she managed to calm down.

Hamed was proud of the Persian civilisation and history, and missed the good, beautiful Iran under the rule of the Shah. Although he was disappointed at what had been happening in Iran since the Islamic government came to power, he never lost hope that Iran would one day be liberated and become a liberal country again.

Calmer, but still trapped in the torturous thoughts of past experiences, Shiva returned to the table. Hamed was oblivious to what he might have said that made her so uncomfortable. He lifted his face away from the *San Francisco Chronicle* and looked at Shiva as she sank into the chair and hung her purse on its back.

"I'm sorry, the restroom was so busy," Shiva apologised and grinned. She had no choice but to stretch her face and maintain a polite smile.

"It's alright. Are you feeling okay?" Hamed asked, as he took off his eyeglasses.

"Oh yes, I'm alright, thanks," She answered, smoothing down her blouse.

As he folded back the newspaper he said, "This is a good article about the presidential elections, if you're interested."

"I'm not interested. In fact, I'm not into politics," Shiva went on again, "I don't believe politicians. Governments start wars, and then sell weapons. They market products that cause diseases, and then sell drugs. It's all about making money." She ran a hand through her hair.

"You're not wrong about corruption, but diseases aren't spread intentionally — just mismanaged," Dr. Salehi said, but Shiva did not seem to be listening.

She continued, "This world is a huge game of chess, in which we are the insignificant white and black pieces, being moved around or removed altogether by bigger hands." Shiva gave a bitter laugh.

The waitress interrupted the heated discussion with the mouth-watering aroma of the dishes she brought to the table. She placed a well-done sizzling steak with mashed potatoes and grilled vegetables in front of Hamed, and served Shiva a Cobb salad with grilled chicken breast. They started eating, and Hamed asked if she wanted to try his steak. She thanked him, saying no. Hamed appreciated that silent break, pretending to focus on the food and talking about how good it tasted.

Trying to keep a decent smile on their faces, they both thought how looks could be deceiving and first impressions might not necessarily last. Shiva glanced at a big advertisement on the front page of the newspaper that Hamed had put aside. A big white cross was on top, and beside it stood a smiling priest. "Donate to help the needy", the advertisement of the charity organisation said. She recalled seeing similar posters on the streets of Tehran; the only difference was a photo of an Imam instead. Next to the advertisement was a long article on the Republican candidate, running for USA President, *Lower Corporate Tax for Big Businesses,* the headline stated. She resumed the conversation.

"Growing up, I always found it funny that those men of religion constantly ask people to give to the poor." She grinned, pointing at the newspaper. "Although they also say that God created all people equal. So why should there be poor people in the first place? Aren't they contradicting themselves?" She added dressing to her salad.

"People were created equal, yes, in the eyes of God, but at the end of the day, it is normal in any society that there are the poor and the rich." He squared his shoulders.

"This is what aristocracy, imperialism, and now extreme capitalism want people to believe. God didn't create the poor; mankind created poverty through their greed and injustice. They want society to be divided into two classes: the few wealthy who own everything and those who work for them." She countered.

"But capitalism aims at vitalising the economy and creating jobs." He spread some butter on a bun.

"Unfortunately, these days capitalism has reached scary stages, even in the developed countries in the West, leading to social inequality." She drank some orange juice.

"But socialism can also be unfair, and the world has realised its danger." He twisted the pepper grinder over his steak.

"The far left doesn't exist in the developed world any longer; it's all centre-left now. Yet, those on the right side of the spectrum still want to go to the farther right; they forgot its danger. They need to reread the history. I wonder why we can't meet in the middle." Shiva gave a wry smile.

As they ate, Shiva talked to Hamed about the Mental Health Week and the main topics that were covered. A psychiatrist and a psychologist could easily get absorbed in a long discussion about mental illness and psychological disorders. They shared interesting points of view, and surprisingly, they did not disagree. "It always starts with a thought in the mind that influences the mood, which affects the chemistry of the brain," Shiva reflected.

"In genetic cases, however, it could start with the chemicals in the brain that affect the mood, and consequently influence the thoughts," he concluded.

They continued eating, feeling more at ease than they were at the beginning. Yet they both sensed that neither of them was what the other was looking for. They finished their dinner and asked for the bill. When the waitress came with two separate ones, Shiva quickly took hers and gave the waitress her Master Card. Hamed did not mind any longer. After all, Shiva was too independent for him. They both knew there would not be a next time. Neither of them regretted that they had met, though. Perhaps they could be good friends. They said goodbye, and Shiva drove home.

The car soared up and dived down the hilly streets of San Francisco, as Shiva reflected. She was glad that she had finally agreed to meet Dr. Salehi. At least, now she knew he was not the one. *I wasn't in my best mood today,* she regretted. She knew that Hamed was a kind person, but the connection between him and all her memories about Iran was inevitable.

Since Shiva had left Iran, she had only visited once to see her parents before they had passed away ten years earlier. Except for her childhood and adolescence — when Iran was a liberal, developed country — she did not have good memories. She was in college when the Iranian revolution erupted. Shiva and her generation participated in the protests, hoping to make their country better, not only for the wealthy but for everyone, not realising that another power would take over and make it worse for all. She had been arrested for possessing French literature books in her bedroom, books believed to be against the Islamic authorities. She had been tortured in prison to tell on other students and released after several months.

She had no one left in Iran to visit. Her only brother had been arrested and tortured to death for a similar reason. After the revolution, Iran had become a huge prison for all Iranians who did not support the regime. She had abandoned Iran, searching for freedom, and since then, she had not welcomed any opportunity that might remind her of that jail.

Her tears streamed down her cheeks as she recalled her brother's memory and her mother's sorrowful eyes. She realised how much she missed them, and she was tired of being alone. Shiva knew she needed someone in her life, but it was not going to be Hamed.

The sunset scene by the water was comforting, yet she couldn't think about anything but having to find another apartment by the end of the month. She had been looking for five weeks. She was getting stressed just thinking about it. Exhausted after a long day that ended with such a challenging date, she at last arrived in her apartment.

While she was sorting out the mail in the kitchen, the phone rang. The caller ID indicated 'Liam MacArthur'. She picked the phone up, "Hi Liam. I've tried to call you many times lately. I was getting worried."

"I'm okay, Mom. Just busy," he said. It was a quick call. She was glad he was alright. She looked at Liam's picture beside his brother's, on the bookshelves. Although it was hard to live far away from her sons, she had insisted on staying in San Francisco after their move to Florida many years earlier.

She walked into the cluttered living room. She cleared away the boxes and suitcases she had prepared for packing and went to her bedroom. The warm air came through the window, as she looked around at every corner of the room that she was going to miss. Shiva moved the pile of clothes from the chair to the bed and closed the window to quiet the noise. With her eyes focused on the sun setting on the ocean in the tableau in front of her, she disconnected from the world and silenced her mind, concentrating on her in-and-out breathing.

Gradually, she left the room for a blissful green place, where she would put her body and mind on hiatus, while letting her soul flutter and breathe some positive energy. She struggled to stop the thoughts jumping up and down — like monkeys — in her head. When she finally let her conscious return to the room, the clock on the wall indicated that an hour had passed. To her, it only felt like a few minutes. She opened the window again to let a breeze in.

Getting ready to sleep, she put the pile of clothes back on the chair and noticed a voice message on the answering machine. She pressed the button, "Hello, this is Steve Johnston, returning your call about the basement suite in my house. It's still available. Give me a call, so we can arrange a time for you to come and have a look. The house is walking distance from the Bay. The rent is reasonable. There's a separate entrance to the basement, so you'll have all the privacy you need. The house is quiet. I live alone." Shiva wrote down his phone number and closed her eyes to sleep.

Despair

She came home after a long day at work, to that splendid house, empty of everything but discomfort. She felt suffocated inside, as if it was even empty of air. The house felt deadly; the girls were in their rooms, most likely reading or talking to their friends on the phone. The doors of their rooms were closed, as usual. The loud snoring approached from the family room. Vincent was on the couch, dozing. Since he had been let go from his work months earlier, his insomnia had been worse than ever.

In desperate need of fresh air, she opened the back door and stepped out to the patio. She did not mind the cold wind. All she needed was to inhale some oxygen, enough to fill up her lungs until the next morning, when she would leave the house again. Looking at the neglected backyard made her feel more heartsick.

"When you have cancer, you either fight it or wait to die." Sophie could not get these words out of her head; they had been screaming at her since she had heard them from Adam. She had not been diagnosed with cancer; she wished! She had been living in this cancer-like nightmare for years. The moment she entered her home, she could not help feeling her life was a meaningless story. Who said there was no place like home? Home could be hell if it had no hope.

All summer, she had deliberately avoided looking at her deserted garden, which used to be her little paradise. Over the past years, she had spent long hours in the summertime — gardening, weeding, and watering her plants. She had planted a precious collection of perennial bushes and shrubs, now being killed by the growing weeds around them. Her lilacs and roses were drying up. Her phlox and dahlias were fading away. Her daisies and peonies were choking. By now, the dead yellow leaves were all over the brown grass, and soon everything would be covered with snow until spring.

She went inside to the kitchen, not feeling hungry, or rather having no appetite to eat. She looked indifferently at the sink which was full of dirty pots, pans, cups, and plates. She groaned. She had just cleaned the kitchen and washed all the dishes the previous night before going to bed. She battled her way among boxes of books, piles of files and binders, heaps of papers and magazines, plastic bags full of items that she had not bought, did not need, and would never use.

Oh God! He bought more stuff. She wanted to scream but felt a lump in her throat. She had recently spent weeks, organising and de-cluttering. She had made several trips to different stores to return whatever she could find a receipt for. She had just dropped off three big donation bags on her way to work. Now the clutter filled every corner of the house once more. *It's about time I closed this joint bank account,* she reminded herself. She ignored all the mess and went to the girls' rooms. "Did you eat?" she asked.

"Yes, we ate at McDonald's," they answered. She said good night and went to her room.

Sophie felt doomed for life with no way out, as if she was locked up in a dark room that had no exit — no door to escape, no window to let in some light. *Only death could save her from this prison* she thought. Her only relief was to sleep; being able to temporarily disconnect from reality was the one single outlet from her daily torment.

Some mornings, she opened her eyes, thinking, *I'm tired of life. Why do I have to wake up? Let me sleep forever. I want to rest in peace.* She was not brave enough to quit; nor was she strong enough to continue, so she waited for a miracle to save her — even a fire to destroy the house and end her life.

She lay in her bed, asking herself why she had waited all these years. For how long would she keep pressing the snooze button and continue sleeping? She was not getting any younger, and the years were slipping by. Why could she not do what she had been thinking of for the last few years? Was it guilt? Fear? Or rather despair? She was so hopeless that her only hope in life was to die — as she was slowly fading away.

The next morning, she woke up to the blaring TV in the family room downstairs, mixed with the loud sound of Vincent's snoring. He had fallen asleep on the couch while watching TV all night. She was determined not to let any of this upset her. She woke up with a great deal of energy and unusual bravery.

She was relieved to know that Vincent was asleep. She showered, got dressed, and woke her daughters as quickly as possible. She panicked when she went to the kitchen and saw five candles on the counter, melting beside some plastic containers. It was not the first time that Vincent had lit candles and left them unattended in the middle of the night. Instead of screaming, she decided to release this negative energy by quietly blowing out the candles.

She tiptoed not to wake him up. She knew that although he had been awake all night, he would doze only for an hour, get up and go out shopping all day. Going out through the front door, she heard him asking, "Sophie, have you prepared the documents for my new business?

Can you please take them to the accountant on your way to work?"

They left, and Vincent stayed on the couch, thinking nobody wanted to help him. *Why is she so mean to me?* he wondered. *I never harm her. What else do they want from me? I pay the bills; I buy everything for them,* he thought. *No one respects me.* Many irrelevant topics crowded his brain.

Vincent was once a geologist in a high-paying profession. Sophie was thankful for the abundant life he offered, but money was not all she needed. Money had no real value for Sophie; her needs were basic, and she was easily satisfied. All she wished for was a peaceful, secure life, a clean, uncluttered home, and someone to share their responsibilities with her. Now that he had lost his job, her fear grew, considering the debts into which he could get himself and her.

With difficulty Vincent tried to lift his overweight body and stand up. He looked in many plastic bags on the coffee table — full of electronics, musical instruments, clothes, books, and kitchenware he had bought over the previous nights. He checked every single item and left them scattered on the floor; receipts of over $500 each were carelessly thrown on the coffee table.

He walked to the chaotic kitchen and opened the fridge to make something to eat, but he did not find one clean pan. Half of the pots and pans he had used were dirty in the sink, and half of them were still on the stove, filled with food he had cooked the previous day, but no one ate. Walking to the bedroom, he tripped over some boxes on the floor. *Damn it!* he raged. He put some clothes on, grabbed his car keys, and left to eat out.

Sophie dropped the girls off at the bus stop, making sure they had enough lunch money, and drove off to work. On the way, she stopped by Tim Horton's to get her morning coffee. She needed to wake herself up. Driving along the busy streets, she thought of Adam. Hopeful sparks brought about some cheer to her face.

She had met Adam a month earlier. He had moved to Quebec City from Toronto for a couple of months to do some research for his work project on French architecture in North America. Sophie worked at the Musée de l'Amérique Francophone; a translator, she had worked on some historical documents for Adam's project. He barely knew anybody in Quebec and was thankful to have found someone to talk to like Sophie.

The first time he had spoken to her, Adam knew it would not be the last. He was puzzled by Sophie's noticeable yet neglected beauty and her passionate, yet indifferent eyes. To him, she seemed like a fading flower, still spreading delightful fragrance. He discovered many conflicting traits that made him curious to explore her.

Her mysteriousness was a riddle for him to solve and a perplexing book to read. He was impressed by her caring nature for her work and her clients, but he was shocked at some comments she made about life, and how she did not care for things in which many other women her age would be interested.

"I always feel heavy pain when I look in your eyes," Adam revealed to her later.

"Living with a depressed person eventually turns you into one," she answered.

"I'm so sorry to hear that, Sophie, but there's always hope," Adam said.

"People only give up on something, after they've tried everything they could." She gave a bitter smile. "Trust me; I wasn't like this fifteen years ago. I've tried everything I could." Her voice cracked.

"Mental illness is a beast stealing the light from the days. It destroys not only the lives of those who suffer from the illness, but also, and more seriously, the lives of those who are around them," Adam agonised, letting out an aching sigh.

"Especially when they refuse to admit their illness or treat it," Sophie added.

"Even when they admit it and receive treatment," Adam said, "those whose lives are connected to the ill person suffer more than he or she does. I know exactly what you mean. I grew up with a sister who suffered from schizophrenia."

"I'm so sorry," Sophie sympathised.

"That was the main reason I didn't want to have children, although I know I'd make a good father," he said.

Adam came into her life like a shady oasis in a barren desert. Sophie found someone who could understand and relate to what she was going through. He grew attached to her, even though he was not sure of the nature of his own feelings. He believed he had shown up in her life at that particular moment for a reason. Even if that reason was only to motivate her to live a life that she deserved, he was content with that small role.

Their roads had crossed at this turning point, leading each to hidden paths. Adam was rethinking his whole career as an architect, wondering if that was what he wanted to do for the rest of his life. Sophie confronted this difficult decision that she had been unable to make for years. Perhaps the midlife crisis that each faced was what brought them closer.

She arrived at the office. Her colleagues noticed that she looked more vibrant than usual. She wore a teal outfit, which reflected the same colour of her eyes and matched her tanned blonde hair. She went to Suzette's office and shut the door behind her.

"I've made my decision." Sophie raised her chin; her emerald earrings glimmered.

"What decision?" Suzette wondered.

"I'm seeking a divorce. I'll talk to him tonight." Sophie sat straighter and folded her arms.

"Will you this time, Sophie? You've been saying this for years." Suzette looked her in the eye.

"I know I've said it many times before, but this time is different. This time, I've found a reason to live for. My children need a healthier, more hopeful mother." Sophie rose from her seat and left.

Sophie went to her office. She checked three voice messages on her office phone — one was from Vincent. He had called and left a message yelling that his life was unbearable, blaming her for all his miseries, and harassing her in various ways. She received his attacks, as she always had, with passive panic, reminding herself that it was just an episode, and it would end in a matter of weeks. She felt the need to scream, cry, but there were no tears left.

Save the good memories and let go, she said to herself. Sophie had given up on this relationship, but why should she give up on life? Why would she spend her remaining days waiting for death, while there was so much in life to enjoy? She recalled everything she had tried, to help Vincent since day one.

Not only had he refused the diagnosis and treatment, but he had also turned against her, considering her his enemy. Refusing to let people who cared for him help out, Vincent gave in to the claws of hopeless depression — ruining his life and the lives of his loved ones, resisting in vain through episodes of manic hyperactivity.

"No one can help you if you don't want to help yourself," she had said to Vincent a couple of years earlier. Over the years, she had carried the two-handled basket of their marriage by herself; now the basket was broken, losing everything it held. She could not save it by herself. Caving in, Sophie would either implode, silently vanishing inside, or explode, emotionally harming herself and Vincent.

It was a chilly autumn day. From the window in her office, Sophie watched the perplexing colours of the trees. She listened to the soothing sound of the wind, playing with the yellow leaves on the pavement. She caught a glimpse of the St. Lawrence River, losing its blueness in the dominant orange of the bigger scene. She smelt winter coming, but this time, she did not fear it. For the first time, winter was not dreadful because she was only thinking about the spring that would follow.

It was almost 4:30 in the afternoon; she left her office and went to see Adam. Feeling the warmth of each other, they enjoyed walking by the river in the cold evening. They went to a small cafe for some crepes and hot chocolate. Sophie stayed silent for a while, staring at something in the air Adam could not spot. He looked at her crumbling eyes and gently asked, "What's wrong Sophie?"

"I'm discouraged again," she answered, twisting her emerald ring. "I'm scared of the unknown."

"You'll live one day at a time," he said.

"Of loneliness." She hugged herself.

"You'll always have yourself." Adam leaned forward.

"I'm not sure I have the courage to tell him." She pressed a hand to her throat.

"No one can force you to continue a life that kills everything beautiful in you." Adam placed his hand on hers.

"It's going to be too complicated." She shook her head.

"Sometimes we stress out over things that end up not happening." He kept eye contact.

"And the guilt!" Sophie covered her eyes with her shivering hands.

"You may be doing him a favour," Adam said.

"I do care for him, but he'll never understand," Sophie groaned.

"One day, he will, when the days prove that you won't harm him in any way."

"I feel sorry for him. I know he caused much damage, but he didn't hurt me on purpose," she cried.

"Mental illness should never be an excuse for abusive behaviour. Sophie, you've tried for years to accept what you can't change. It's about time you changed what you can't accept," he said, looking her in the eye.

"I feel sorry for my children," said Sophie, tears rolling down her face.

"Your children will be happier when they live with a happier mother."

"Yes, I know; they know and understand everything." She rubbed her shoulder.

"Sophie, you're an intelligent and strong woman. You're young and beautiful. You deserve to live. When logic tells you it will get worse, it will only get worse. Don't hold on tight to fake hope; you're only wasting your life. Do something now! Don't wait until the day when you say to yourself, 'I wish I'd started years ago'."

"It's so painful," she sobbed.

"No one said healing was painless," said Adam; "we only heal through the pain."

"He'll complicate everything for me; it'll take years." She turned her face away.

"Years are passing anyway, so you better start now!" Adam firmly said.

Sophie had many contradictory emotions churning inside her; regret was not one of them. Her conversation with Adam felt like an internal rush of thoughts. He knew how to restore her lost faith. It was getting late, and it was time to go home. Adam gave her a warm hug, and he let his fingers go gently through her soft hair. He whispered in her ear, "Everything will be alright. You're not the first one to go through this, and you won't be the last." His words sparked a gleam of life in her body. They walked back to where she had parked her car and said goodbye.

Sophie took her car and drove back. It was dark, and the streets were noiseless. There were hardly any people walking. Sophie thought about her two daughters. She did not want them to be harshly neglected like the poor flowers in her garden. She wanted to be stronger and happier for them. She was determined to talk to Vincent that night.

She enjoyed the drive, listening to songs in her warm car. She visualized her own small house, the one she had always dreamed of. She remembered her old plan to do her Masters degree in communications and decided to pass by TÉLUQ University the following day to inquire about distance education programs. She was full of hope and at peace. Close to home, a speeding truck suddenly crossed in front of her. Sophie slammed on the brakes — but she could not stop the car.

Time Heals

She sat at the dresser in front of the mirror, putting on her jewellery and finishing the last touches of her makeup. Dressed in a long white gown, she looked at her reflection — a tall curvy young lady, whose dark brown eyes shone with radiance. The contrast between her elegant white dress and her glowing dark chocolate skin created a mysterious harmony, matching her eyes — the nearly black iris surrounded by white.

She wore dangling diamond earrings and celestial perfume. Her thick black hair was braided into hundreds of thin plaits and made into a round bun underneath a long white tulle veil that reached the floor when she stood up. It was her wedding day; the ceremony was in two hours. Scatter-brained, she glanced in the mirror, not at her face, but rather at a framed photo on the opposite wall of a young lady and a two-year-old girl. The girl looked like a miniature of the mother.

Her gaze turned to the quote "The present moment is all we have." Hand-written in capital letters on thick white paper, it hung under a wide picture of colourful galaxies of countless stars on the grey wall above her desk. She stared at the bookshelves around the desk, as if she did not want to say goodbye to anything in her room. She picked up a thick book on her desk — Endless Cosmos.

She almost heard her mother's voice talking with her, recalling a famous conversation between them, of which her father repeatedly reminded her as she grew up. Once when she was not even four years old, she asked her mother on their way home from church, "Who made God?"

Her mother answered, "God made everything, honey. He's the Creator."

"But who made God?" She repeated her question.

"God's been there since forever," her mother explained.

"But who made God?" Julia asked again.

Giving up on finding an answer that might satisfy her curious daughter, her mother said, "Maybe you should ask him."

But Julia did not stop there; instead, she asked, "Why is God he, not she?"

Her mother giggled. "You're such a genius, pretty little girl," she said, holding her tight and feeling proud of her brilliant daughter.

Her mother encouraged her to ask questions, even when she did not have answers for her. "Half of the answer is in the question," she had always said to Julia. Michelle was a successful lawyer and a brilliant young lady who was loyal to her career without neglecting her family and home. She dedicated every minute away from work to her daughter and her husband.

Julia was alone in her room; Gaby, her friend since kindergarten, had left half an hour earlier in order to supervise many preparations for the ceremony in the church. Still absorbed in her thoughts, Julia heard a familiar knock on the door. Knowing very well who it was, she smiled and said, "Come in, Dad." She turned around and looked at the door, while it was opening.

"Hello Ms. Brown, my beautiful princess. Let me get enough of you before you become Mrs. Smith soon." He came in.

"Dad," she said, looking up, "I'll always be your little girl." She spread her arms wide.

"I know, dear. I know. But you'll be missed in this house." He grabbed her right hand and kissed it, as she rose from her seat.

"Dad, I'm worried about you." She pressed her hands to his arms. "Please consider moving to Washington. Give it another thought."

"Honey, I'll be fine. Don't worry about me. I just want to see you one of the most prosperous women in this world, as your mother was." He drew in a long breath.

"I wish she was here today," Julia agonised.

Thomas' voice cracked, and tears brightened his big eyes. He turned around and covered his kind dark face with his right hand, looking through his long fingers at the picture of Michelle and Julia on the wall. He wiped his tears while looking the other way, then turned to Julia and smiled. "The best I can do is to tell you what your mother would have told you on your wedding day," Thomas said.

"Tell me, please." Julia tilted her head to one side while listening.

"To fall in love and find your other half is a fantastic feeling; to have a home and family of your own gives your life an immense satisfaction. But don't let any of this make you forget yourself, your career, and your passion. You're always more important. If you don't take care of yourself, you won't be able to give them what they need or deserve." Thomas grinned.

"I'll try my best," Julia promised.

"Now, it's time for the beautiful bride to get ready; people are waiting for you. While you'll be walking down the aisle, remember that your mother is right there watching over you and is very proud of you."

The last time Julia had seen her mother, they were at home baking gingerbread cookies together. Michelle, realising there were not enough eggs, had driven to the nearest grocery store to buy some. In a horrific car accident, she had died, leaving her five-year-old girl to her husband. Julia had waited forever to taste the bittersweet cookies which were never baked, and from that moment on, smelling ginger and cinnamon made her feel sick.

Thomas turned to steal a last look at his daughter before leaving the room. Although his wound had been gradually healing over the years, it felt fresh and bleeding anew. Julia's eyes had hardly any tears. She had seldom shed tears since the day of her mother's death, as if all her tears had been generously poured out that day, leaving no more.

Thomas lived the rest of his years for his daughter on the memories he shared of her mother — the love of his life. He lived for Julia, for she was the only reason left for him to live. A prestigious prosecutor at the Department of Justice in Texas, he could always find the time to spend with his daughter in spite of his extremely busy schedule.

Growing up, Julia heard him tell many stories of when her mother was still alive and conversations between them when Julia was little. He always talked to her about Michelle and told her stories of how they had fallen in love when they were teenagers, and how their love grew more powerful and secure through the years.

Julia still had a vivid picture of her mother after all the years, and around this memory were many contradictory thoughts in her head. She yearned passionately for her mother's presence on that day. And though she felt heartbroken about leaving her father alone, she felt blessed and thankful to have found David.

It was time to go to the church. A white limousine, simply decorated with blue ribbons and pink roses, waited in front of the house. Julia had tried to convince her father several times that there was no need for a limousine for only the two of them, but he had insisted. After all, she was his only daughter, and he happily wanted to do everything he could to make her special day the best possible, so he would see Michelle happy and satisfied in his dreams.

The limo drove Julia and her father to the church of the Holy Trinity where the ceremony was about to take place. It was a sunny, yet cool winter day, and the humidity filled the air. On the way, the driver played classical music that took Thomas years back to his own wedding day. He smelt Michelle standing next to him in front of the altar.

Looking through the opposite window, Julia was eager to see David. When the vehicle passed by the University of Houston, she recalled the first day David had ever approached her after months of admiring her from afar. She had been working on her master's degree. He always saw her around in the department talking with her supervisor. He often heard Dr. Lagrange talking about how caring Julia was as a person, and how smart as a student. Yet one of David's students, who happened to take one class with Julia, referred to her as a cold, snobbish girl when David mentioned her name in one of their conversations. Hearing different opinions about her, David grew curious to know more about her intriguing personality.

One afternoon, he stopped by the library to collect some books he had requested. She was there, writing an assignment in the far corner at a small table by the window. He could not help getting closer; he tried to approach her, asking if she had finished with one of the books in front of her because one of his students was looking for it. "Hello Dr. Smith, I've almost finished the book," she replied, "I'm returning it at the end of the day."

Then he started a conversation about her research. It was her final project in her master's degree. Knowing that she was planning on starting her PhD soon after, he asked, "What is your PhD thesis going to be about?"

"Spacetime," she answered.

David stared at her with cow eyes. "I'm writing a paper on spacetime for a conference that I'm going to present in the spring," he said. They talked. He told her how Dr. Lagrange spoke very highly of her. David asked Julia to come and talk to him in his office the following day to discuss if he could supervise her PhD.

The next day, they met in his office and talked about her graduate study. They discussed her thesis topic, what made her choose it, and her plans for her research. They considered what science had discovered so far about gravity and relativity. Julia was surprised that she opened up to him comfortably. Curious to know more about her, David turned the conversation to another dimension. He said, "You chose a promising thesis, Julia. Time is a very interesting topic. It's funny because I've always been obsessed with time, all my life." He grinned and ran his fingers through his ash brown hair.

"Me too. My father reminds me every now and then of a question I kept asking when I was in Kindergarten. I asked why the hour was 60 minutes and not 100 minutes," Julia giggled.

"You started very early," he said, "I remember when I was in junior high, I argued with my science teacher that similar to space with its three known dimensions, maybe past, present, and future were the three dimensions of time that we know of or rather created in our minds. I continued arguing that if time could go forward, we could also make it go backward." He crossed his arms over his chest.

"I know," Julia agreed. "Where did the difference between past and future come from?" she wondered.

"Time is a concept that humans created," David reflected. "I often feel this whole world might be just an illusion." He sat straight and smoothed his shirt.

"Truth is a myth. Everything is perception. The way time seems to us on Earth is very different from how it seems somewhere else in the galaxy, never mind the rest of the universe. I find it mind blowing that at certain spots in the cosmos, time completely stops."

"I find it eye opening," he replied. "Sometimes I wonder if a black hole is what some people call Hell. Or if the big bang is just another scientific term for creation," David wondered, hands gripping onto some papers on the desk.

"The only way out of a black hole is through it, by keeping a steady speed at a certain distance from the centre on its boundary, where one crosses over to worlds of new dimensions," Julia said. "Perhaps we must go through Hell first in order to reach Heaven at last." Julia rested her chin in her palm.

"That's philosophical," David said. His pupils dilated. Staring at Julia's wide eyes, he continued, "We're so ignorant of the universe we live in, Julia. Exactly, as we're oblivious to our human psyche deep inside." David leaned back in his chair.

Julia was thankful that he accepted to supervise her PhD thesis. They scheduled several meetings to discuss the Research plan. He got to know much more about her.

David was attracted not only to her academic genius in physics, but also her emotional intelligence in human relations, contrary to what some people may have thought. Some people mistook her quietness and shyness as being aloof and unfriendly. But those who knew her closely felt her thoughtfulness and compassion.

Julia and David were as opposite as night and day, not only in their skin colour, but also in their personalities; yet they were united by one mission. A positive extrovert, he saw the world as a dynamic place, full of good-hearted people, who had so much to give. What Julia loved the most about him, however, was his ability to see the strengths in others, and surely he saw her strengths and beauty.

Day after day, he became accustomed to seeing her, talking to her, and listening to her brilliant questions and funny comments. Only one week after she defended her thesis, and coincidentally or intentionally, on her twenty-fifth birthday, David proposed. Julia barely needed time to think. They had known each other and worked together for two years, which felt like living temporarily in Heaven. He was the right partner with whom to discover her path to the cosmos and find answers to her countless questions.

Yet, again, life refused to grant Julia complete happiness. Three months later, and only seven weeks before their wedding, David had received a prestigious job offer at NASA headquarters in Washington DC. The day she heard about this, her world collapsed. She could not comprehend the possibility of leaving her father in Houston. She asked David for a few days to think it over, and he was patient enough to give her all the time she needed. He understood the strong ties between Julia and Thomas.

She spent a long time alone in her room reconsidering her whole life, asking if she could ever move away from her father. She knew it was not fair to ask David to sacrifice that opportunity. The most painful choice, however, would be to let David go and cancel their wedding.

The news was bitter for Thomas. Julia was all he had. But he did not want her to lose David, knowing how much David loved and cared for her. Thomas' main wish was to see Julia happy and successful. Nights passed while Thomas and Julia were thinking, aching in silence.

Julia was nearly ready to let David leave alone when Thomas decided they had to talk. Trying to suppress his troubled emotions, Thomas reassured her that she should not worry at all. Julia, on the other hand, tried to convince him to consider moving to Washington, but that was out of the question for him. He could hardly breathe away from that house in Houston, which bore Michelle's scent in every corner.

They talked for hours. "You're going to apply for NASA Pathways Intern Employment Program," Thomas encouraged her. He searched on the NASA website. The deadline to apply was the following day. She emailed her application, and two weeks later she was accepted. It was so fast and smooth that Julia had a feeling it was a sign that she had to continue her life with David.

As the limousine turned onto the street, Julia looked at her father and again battled the torturous thoughts of leaving him. They arrived at the church. All the guests were already seated, waiting for the bride. It was a small wedding; beside the two families, most of the invitees were David's students and friends. The church was decorated with blue ribbons and pink roses, and the golden rays of the tender sun came through the narrow windows, pouring grace on the place. The scent of candles created gentle warmth. While Julia was anxiously looking at this delightful scene from the limo's window, her father got out of the car, opened the door, and helped her out.

Gaby, her maid of honour, dressed in an elegant blue gown and holding a pink rose bouquet, went in first with Joel, David's best man and best friend in a navy-blue suit and a pink tie. Thomas walked side-by-side with Julia, his eyes full of nostalgic tears of joy. Julia's eyes, however, were smiling at David, who was standing impatiently at the other end of the aisle.

Julia's arm was tightly tangled in Thomas', as if she was unwilling to let go of him. They walked slowly to the graceful music, until she was one step away from David; he was still taller than her in her high heels. Thomas left her to her soon-to-be husband and went back to sit in the first row beside David's parents. With lots of paradoxical emotions, he watched the ceremony alongside a flashback of Julia's life since she was born until she became a pretty bride. Michelle was in every scene.

The pastor announced them husband and wife and asked David to kiss the shy bride, as if they hadn't kissed before. They walked as a married couple to the entrance of the church to thank all people individually. Friends and family members stayed to take photos with the bride and groom.

After an hour or so, everyone left except Thomas, Gaby, and David's parents, who had to leave shortly thereafter.

Gaby stayed for a while, talking to the newlyweds. "Promise you'll visit Dad when you can," Julia reminded her for the twentieth time.

"Yes, Julia, please don't worry about him. Enjoy your honeymoon and your new life. I am here for him whenever he needs anything. I promise," Gaby comforted her. She kissed Julia, said goodbye, and left.

It was very hard for Thomas to say goodbye; he wished time would stop at that moment. It was getting dark and chilly, yet their affection kept the three of them warm as the stars brightened the black sky. They felt a few raindrops on their skin. In the cool night breeze, the inexplicable sweet scent, which Thomas knew very well, brought comfort and peace to Julia's soul.

"I'll come visit when you have your first baby. Don't take too long. It better be a girl," Thomas grinned, embracing Julia's hands.

"I'll do my best to make it happen soon, Thomas," David jested. "I want a girl, too. We'll call her 'Joy'."

"No Dad, I'll come see you sooner," Julia disagreed. Thomas held Julia tight in his shaky arms and said goodbye. He stood watching their car until it could no longer be seen. And alone, he went home.

Liberation

She decided to leave before dawn when it was still dark. The dew filled the air and crystallised on the black-hearted scarlet poppies, spattered like blood drops across the olive carpet of grass. The earthy smell barely made it to her nostrils. She dragged her feet across the vast fields, clutching an elegant small gold container in her distressed hands.

She had hardly slept for two nights. How could she let her eyes catch a wink after the death of the one person who had transformed her entire life and changed her views of the world? Lost in the void, her frozen eyes did not need to look at the way ahead; her feet knew it by heart — the way they had walked behind his dead body to the tomb hours earlier. She came very early, before the sun rose on the Town of Peace with her spices and ointments.

Her whole world had turned into a huge abyss since she had witnessed his horrific execution. Her heart was bleeding, wounded by the dagger of betrayal and injustice. What she had experienced was beyond comprehension; she could hardly picture how her life would be without him.

For many years, her days and nights had revolved around him. She accompanied him wherever he went and listened to every word he said. Their conversations opened her eyes to things that were hidden; her heart, to values that were lost; and her mind, to truths that were covered by hatred and resentment.

Three years earlier, Marab had decided to go out for a walk on a hot summer day, to breathe fresh air; she was suffocating at home. She walked alone, avoiding any chance to raise eyes, lest she should meet someone else's gaze. Although she hid her face with her long dark scarf, some children recognised her. They followed her and loudly sang humiliating songs, calling her 'adulterous', throwing stones at her.

Strayed and broken, she walked aimlessly as she contemplated her whole life. Marab was emotionally abused, mentally messed-up, and spiritually disoriented. She walked away from her house until she reached the shore of the Great Lake. Looking at the pristine water, she wished she could hide herself under the waves forever. She stood by the shore for a long time until she noticed a large crowd gathering around someone. She walked toward them, away from the lake.

As much as she avoided crowds, she could not resist coming closer to get a clearer view of the man and to hear what he was saying. While squeezing through the congregation, her large scarf fell and rested on her elbows. She was not concerned that her face was recognised. Ignoring the insulting words people were saying to her, she made her way among them to find a seat close to the preacher.

She was lost in his indescribable eyes, when he said, "Questioning your faith will never weaken it; it will strengthen it. Doubt is usually the first step toward certainty. Questioning your beliefs will benefit you more than following traditions. Your religious leaders don't know about the Eternal any more than you do. They shut the gates of heaven against people, hide the keys to knowledge and substitute them with half-truths. When a blind leads a blind, they both fall."

Many people in the crowd, who recognised Marab's face, were surprised that she was sitting there with them. They were whispering among themselves, wondering what

Marab — the possessed woman — was doing there. Some of them moved away from her, lest they should be haunted by the demons inside her.

Marab, an only child, lived in her parents' house and had enough money for her expenses without the need to work. Unmarried and childless, she lived by herself after her parents had died and spent her empty days and long nights, isolated from a society that did not accept her.

"Even when you deny the Truth," the teacher continued, looking up, "you will end up finding the Truth. But when your faith is shaky, tepid, and bland, you aren't achieving anything or reaching anywhere. The Supreme isn't far from you. Look inward. You — body, mind, and soul — are but a miniature of the whole Universe. You're a miracle of creation. When you know yourself, you'll know everything."

Marab's life was so purposeless — all she did was eat and sleep. She ate without stopping to the point that she was never hungry, yet she would still eat more. Her constant cravings made it impossible for her to ever feel satisfied; and her laziness eliminated all motivation for any activity.

"The kingdom of heaven is here and now," he proclaimed, palms up. "Look around. Nature is the most inspirational sacred text to read. The Creator speaks through creation. The Highest doesn't dwell in temples built by hands. The Divine abides within you."

Although Marab lived in abundance and had more than she needed, she did not share or give; she greedily wanted more. She was always scared of losing what she had, thinking it was never enough. Insecure, she always lived in fear. Her inflated pride built high walls around her, disconnecting her from people. She despised them; they detested her.

"Seek the truth so that you can see the Almighty during your mortal life," the preacher went on. "Don't be afraid to deviate when searching your way. You'll find your own secret path, leading you to the Truth," he reassured.

Marab was always thirsty for attention and acceptance — through short-lived relationships that never satisfied her hunger for love. Her fiery lust never faded away; but every time she knew a man, she despised herself because none of them gave her the respect or appreciation she yearned for. All men treated her the same way — with a flaming desire at first, only to abandon her at the end.

"The only commandment I give you is love. If you have all the knowledge and faith but no love, there's no benefit to your soul." The preacher rose and walked among people, talking to them individually. Marab felt uncomfortable, thinking that he might come closer to talk to her. She made her way up and through the large number of people. She walked to the shore until they finished eating.

In her community, Marab was loathed and looked down upon, feared by children and many adults as well. She envied those who, although much poorer and needier, enjoyed simple blessings she did not have. In spite of being rich, healthy and pretty, she felt emptiness.

Bitter and lonely, she lived in worry and uncertainty. Her beauty was hidden by her ugly wrath and excessive pride; her sloth and gluttony gradually ruined her well-being; her greed and envy amplified her sense of deprivation; and her lust caused her to loathe herself and to be scorned by others.

Marab stared at the master from a distance, amazed at his preaching. She had not gone to the house of worship for years since the last time, as a teenager, she criticised by people for not being married like most girls her age. But this person's teaching was different from that of the preachers at the Temple. He explained things she had thought about, and answered questions she had always asked. His sermon was profound and powerful, addressing both her mind and soul.

Unaware that she was communicating with people, she asked a man passing by, "Who is this person?"

"Are you not from here?" the man asked, head tilted. "This is Yesham. He came from a small town in the North, and now he's known in many cities in the province."

In order to get a better view and reach hearing distance, she squeezed herself through the crowd, until she came to the very first row right across from him. Looking in his large eyes, she was absorbed by an inexplicable magnetism toward the mysterious secrets hidden in them. Listening to his gripping voice, she was captivated by the wisdom flowing from his mouth. Curiously checking every inch of his face and body, she concentrated on what he was saying.

"Don't judge others," he said, "thinking you'll never do what they do. You never know what may come across your life and make you do the very same thing you're judging them for. You have no excuse. When you judge someone else, you're condemning yourself."

Staring down, Yesham drew figures and letters with his forefinger in the sand. After a while, he looked around, broke the silence and continued, "The true salvation for your soul is to free your mind from resentment and revenge, to liberate your heart from hatred and envy, to overcome your worries and fears, to conquer your weaknesses and flaws, to live in gratitude and contentment, to beat darkness with light, to defeat despair with hope, and to eventually attain your inner peace and eternal comfort."

Yesham ended his sermon and started talking to his mentees, who were sitting around him, while people started leaving one after another. All of a sudden, Marab found herself sitting there alone, a few feet away from him. They both looked at each other for a long time. For some reason, unknown to her, she was unable to move her body; her brain froze up, and her eyes were fixed on his.

At last, he stood up and walked toward her. She rose and waited until he came near. She looked up to his all-knowing eyes, full of compassion, like no one she had seen before. His tender hands touched her arms and hair in a way she had forgotten, for nobody had touched her that way since her mother had died.

He smiled and said, "Why are you afraid? Treat people as you want them to treat you. Don't be scared of them, so they won't be scared of you. If you want them to love you, love them. Forgive them if you want them to forgive you. Don't judge them if you don't want them to judge you, but even if they do, it's their sin, not yours. If you want them to smile at you, smile at them. It works. Try it! It's far simpler than you think."

On her feet still, Marab listened to his words, gazing at his lips in silence. "Give more and expect less," he continued, looking her in the eyes, "don't lose today regretting yesterday or fearing tomorrow. Tomorrow will take care of itself. Live the moment and be content; you'll always find something to be thankful for. Don't let despair darken your way, but rather lighten it with hope — for when there's no hope, there's no life. And life is a gift; make the most of it. I hope to see you again." His wide brown eyes glittered contagious, positive energy.

Yesham left with his devotees, and Marab stood still, trying to fathom what had just happened. A man talked to her with this respect and that much care! For years, people had been avoiding not only talking to her, but even looking at her, let alone touching her. She did not move and stayed still, staring at him for a while after he had left. Going farther, he looked back at her many times with the same mesmerising smile, his black hair floating with the wind around his affectionate face, until he vanished, and she could see him no more.

Looking around in an enjoyable shock, she found herself smiling without knowing it, and she could not understand why. She let her own hands go over the same spots he had touched on her hair, arms, and back. She stayed there alone; the whole shore was completely hers. It was the end of the week, and everybody hurried home, as the day of observance was about to start. Taken by the colours mingling in the sky, she went closer to the water to watch the sunset. She heard the sound of the unceasing waves one after another, enjoying that she had the whole lake to herself. There was nobody around.

Marab took off all her clothes and threw herself utterly naked into the sea, letting the waves carry her body and cover it all up. She felt the warm water on her bare skin and let her long black hair sail behind her body, carried by the soft offshore wind. She washed herself of all the hatred and blame that had lived within her for so long. Floating on the water, her body felt light after shedding the despair and fear she had known for nearly her entire life.

From a distance, she watched the branches of the olive trees dancing with the breath of Mother Nature and listened to them playing the peaceful symphony of her salvation. After a long time — she had no idea how long — she came out of the water. She lay down on the pebbly shore, looking at the dark sky, lightened by innumerable shining stars. The warm breeze tickled her bare skin. The whole of nature was celebrating this moment with her; even the rocks underneath, were soft to her unclothed body, of which she was not ashamed. For the first time, she learned to accept herself as she was, not regretting the past or fearing the future.

When her long mane was dry, she reluctantly decided to leave the blissful scene. She stood up and put on her clothes. As she walked away from the shore, her long scarf slid down her soft hair and was carried by the air, where it stayed behind and was slowly covered by sand. From that moment onward, her comforted, smiling face and glowing large brown eyes told all who saw her that she was a new person.

This turning point — her liberation — was also a moment of revelation. While walking home, Marab recited to herself, "I'd lived long before I was born. I'll last much longer after I die. It's not my choice when I came to Earth, or when I leave. The body I take to be part of this world is mortal, unlike my mind and soul. Many things in my life are not my choices," Marab went on; "my choice is how I decide to respond to them. What matters is maintaining proper relations with the souls around, as well as experiencing the right connection with the origin of all souls in the centre."

"The way I'll spend my afterlife is a continuation of how I live my life here and now. If I succeed in keeping the hope till the end, I'll enjoy the peace, comfort, and freedom of this faith in eternal enlightenment with no sense of time or space. Nevertheless, if I get trapped in despair, I'll live through the self-torment, distress, and regret of this hopelessness, where there will be neither exit nor end," Marab concluded, embracing the air.

She arrived home after a long walk and went to bed. She fell into a deep slumber that she had not experienced for years. She slept in peace until sunrise, when the musical singing of the birds woke her, calling for hope, joy, and freedom. She woke up with an energetic strength that she had not felt all her wasted years of laziness.

She cleaned her house and went through many belongings, most of which she realised she would not need. She prepared piles of things to give away and opened her door to the sun rays and neighbours. She stacked everything in front of her door and stood there, smiling at people passing by.

The neighbourhood children checked what they could take when they heard that she was giving everything away for free. The very same children who stoned her in the past smiled back at her and gave her hugs when they saw her open arms, inviting them. The children ran back to tell their parents, who were speechless with disbelief. Marab at last was not afraid of people, and they no longer feared her.

She decided that she had to look for Yesham and talk to him again. She went out in the green fields, searching for him. She walked around all day, asking everybody she saw if they knew where he was. People were very surprised that she was talking to them, let alone in a kind way.

At last, she saw a crowd, and her heart told her that he was in their midst. Her heart was right. When Yesham turned to her, he said, "I knew you were going to come back."

"I had no choice but to come back," she said. Her hoop gold earrings shimmered, as her eyes gazed at his.

"Good to see you again," he said, eyes widened.

"Thank you for believing in me when I doubted myself. Thank you for restoring my faith in humanity. You're the reason I can smile again," she said, her arms open.

"It makes me happy to see you smile," he responded.

"There's a lot more to learn. I want to listen to what you say, and I have many questions. I want to be with you wherever you go." Thick locks of hair cascaded from under her head scarf.

"I have nothing to offer. I don't have a place to lay my head," he said, arms clasped behind his body.

"You have everything I need, and more." Marab said, hands on chest.

"My way is neither easy nor pleasant." Yesham drew in a deep breath.

"Your way is comforting and eye-opening. I'm ready to travel around with you. I have money; my parents left me a fortune. I'm willing to share this money with you and your followers for food and shelter." She edged closer to him and extended a hand.

Since that day, Marab and Yesham had never been apart. She spent all her time with him and many others, who also followed them and helped with their mission. After having been an outcast for decades, Marab returned to the Temple again. However, going with Yesham was different. Listening to him reading the scriptures and shedding light on their depth formed an exceptional experience for her.

Marab and Yesham grew intimate and often had private conversations. She received the words of wisdom from his mouth and he praised her comprehensive perception. After he had finished a long sermon, she approached him and said, "Sometimes I don't understand you." Her pupils dilated.

"Ask. I love your questions, Marab," he said.

"How could you turn the other cheek if someone slapped you? And why? This is humiliating." Her forehead puckered with disapproval.

"What do you suggest, then? Slap them back?" He answered with a question. Marab remained silent. She twirled her hair and tucked it behind her ear, looking away.

"If I slapped them back," he continued, "both of us would keep fighting until at least one of us, if not both were dead. But if I turned the other cheek and walked away, do you think the other person would slap me again?"

"Maybe not," she shrugged. Marab wished there were fair laws and trustworthy judges in the kingdom.

"It's not so important who started the fight," Yesham said, head lifted. "The question is who will end it? And it takes a lot of strength and wisdom to end a fight." He inhaled a deep breath and blew out slowly.

"Why would I offer to go two miles if I was forced to go only one?" Marab folded her arms; her gold bracelets clinked.

"When you're forced to go one mile, you'll do it, feeling oppressed, but when you offer the extra mile, it will be a favour you're doing that they'll owe you." Yesham propped his elbows on his knees and rested his chin in his palms.

"How can I forgive a person who keeps hurting me over and over again?" Marab asked, narrow-eyed. She rose and walked to the sage plant beside the rock.

"Forgiveness doesn't mean you'll let yourself be hurt by the same person over and over again. Get them out of your life, but hold no grudges or desire for revenge. Understand that they hurt you because they themselves are hurting. Forgiveness is not a favour you do them; it's a favour you do yourself to free it from the pain of resentment. Choose to either hurt or heal." Yesham rose from his seat and paced to another rock.

"It's so hard to love my enemies. It's not even possible," she said, sniffing the sage leaves. She extended a hand with some leaves to Yesham.

"Believe me, Marab, it's much harder to hate them." Yesham turned around and sat on the rock across from her. "When you hate, you harm no one but yourself. Hating someone wastes much of your good energy and turns your own life into Hell, while they don't even remember you exist." He tasted the bitter sage. "But loving your enemies will be easy when you realise that they have their weaknesses, too. They just look at the scene from the opposite angle." The sweet aroma of the sage leaves stuck to Yesham's hand.

"How will transgressors enter the kingdom of heaven before the strict observers of the laws of our religion?" she asked, intrigued. Her garment billowed out around her.

"Sinners, only those who know they are, can hardly judge someone else who also sins," said Yesham, stroking his beard. "They may unintentionally defend them in front of others. While the religious are best at judging. Sinners who believe their sins have been forgiven hold no guilt or grudges. They forgive themselves and others. They heal."

"Sometimes you confuse me," she said, "you preach not to judge, why are you judging the religious, then?" She shook her head; her gold earrings swayed to the sparrows' chirping.

"I don't judge them, dear. I pity only those of them who are preoccupied with man-made rules, too busy to experience the faith the scriptures present. I feel sorry for them because following the laws distracted them from enjoying the depth of the relationship with the Universe. Believing in something doesn't taste as sweet as experiencing it. They don't even know what they're missing," said Yesham, head down.

"They observe the laws of our fathers. They believe this is the right way," Marab argued. She threaded a hand through her wavy hair.

"And by obeying the laws," Yesham explained, "they feel righteous and complete, in no need of grace. They're missing out on the most precious gift of all. Because they think they don't need forgiveness, they can hardly forgive anybody. They judge and look down on those who don't keep the laws, let alone people of different faiths."

"Yesham, I'm worried about you," Marab said, her eyes fixed on his, "It's not wise to confront the priests. Please, leave them alone. Don't make them more enraged than they already are."

"Marab," he replied, holding her arms, "when did you see me confronting them? It's they who confront me. I only respond to them." He rose, smoothed his clothing and walked ahead.

Yesham preached in the houses of worship in every town he passed until he was kicked out by the authorities. People were divided. Many remained in the Temple under the pressure of the Elders — some out of fear, some out of submission, and a few out of satisfaction; yet more followed Yesham to the fields and on the hills.

A large number of people viewed Yesham as a wonder maker; they came from far away to get fed, and to be cured. They glorified him for his god-like traits. On the other hand, some simple people, marginalised by society and rejected by religion for being sinners, traitors, and misfits, went after Yesham, hungry for acceptance and thirsty for inclusion. Some of the oppressed soldiers also came and listened to him and were comforted by his soothing stories. They followed him because he healed their souls before their bodies.

The priests saw Yesham as an alarming danger; they believed he was plotting to lead their subjects to rebel against them. Yesham's teachings did not satisfy their pride. When he called for accepting all people, including those whom they considered enemies, regardless of their tribe, tongue, or belief, it was as if he was speaking to them in a language from another planet. And the more he talked to them about love, the more they hated him.

The King viewed Yesham as a political menace that could cause chaotic unrest in the province and potentially an uprising against the Emperor himself. Listening to the public on the streets talking about Yesham and seeing his followers increase in number by the hour, the soldiers believed he was going to crown himself a king, leading a revolution against the Throne. Rumours spread. Messengers from the royal court were sent to question Yesham asking if he claimed to be the king of his nation. He replied, "My kingdom is not of this world."

It was the Feast of Liberation. Yesham and Marab were in the Temple to celebrate. Many of those, whom he had healed from sickness, came to worship him, but he fled the crowd. They followed him yelling, "O Lord, bless us." Yesham retreated to his secret corner, which nobody knew about except Marab and himself, out of the Temple to hide from the people who ran after him for his blessings.

A league of Elders of the Temple besieged Yesham as he walked out and stopped him. "Do you call yourself God?" the high priest firmly asked. Yesham remained silent. "Do you teach those people that you are their lord and ask them to worship you?" Yesham was questioned again.

"I spoke and taught openly. I said nothing in secret. Go ask those who heard me what I taught them," Yesham replied.

Some fanatics gathered around him picking up stones. He calmly asked, "For what do you stone me?"

They furiously answered, "For blasphemy because you, a mere man, claim to be God."

To which he replied, "Is it not written in your law 'I have said you are gods' ?" The crowds were divided. Some considered Yesham a lunatic, some a heretic. Many believed he was possessed by demons. Others assumed he practised the magic he had learned in the neighbouring lands. They tried to seize him, but he escaped their grasp.

Those who had come to glorify him hours earlier realised there might not be benefits from exalting him any longer. They dismissed from their minds everything Yesham had done for them. His small circle of devotees still believed in him, yet they battled this unbearable inner conflict, fearing arrest.

Marab warned Yesham many times, suggesting that they move somewhere else because she was frightened of losing him. He himself knew that he would eventually be killed. Marab lived in fear until she saw it happening in front of her eyes. At last, Yesham was arrested and sentenced to death. Marab stood before his dying body — humiliatingly and violently executed in front of all by soldiers, one of whom was Marios.

Marios used to be one of the men whom Marab had known years earlier, but when he saw her with Yesham later, he could hardly believe how she was transformed.

Day after day, Marios had grown absorbed in Yesham's sermons and came and listened to his words of comfort. He found the kindness that he had not known before. To Marios and many people who walked his way, Yesham was the only hope they found in an unfair and cruel world that refused and excluded them.

Marios followed Yesham even on the day of his execution, although he was not on duty, when all his followers fled in fear. Standing in the dreadful scene, in the midst of the screaming noise of chaotic crowds, Marab and Marios exchanged silent glances of sorrow and despair. Marios came closer to Marab, held her tight, and sobbed like a child. With tearful eyes, looking up at Yesham, she let Marios pour all his heartache on her shoulders, but her arms were too heavy to hold him. She remained motionless. A furious storm blackened the sky, and the ground was shaken by a raging earthquake. People ran away as Yesham breathed his last.

On her way to the tomb two days after his burial, Marab was still recalling every minute she had spent with Yesham, their memorable conversations, and unforgettable memories, as she walked alone the long way. She pondered how life would be without his inspiring words, soothing eyes, and healing hands. Her feet were painfully sore after having walked for over two hours; she was extremely fatigued and slow.

The hopeful pink rays of the orange sun were slowly cracking the melancholic navy skies, forming a thick purple layer that soon would be turned into merciful blue realms over the peaceful green fields. Realising that the sky was getting brighter, the sparrows came out of their nests, looking for food. They chirped a faithful song, announcing a new day had begun.

She was getting closer to the graveyard. Her heart dropped to the ground when she saw that the stone covering the tomb had been moved away. First, she thought it was her eyes' illusion, being worn out because of excessive crying. But when she looked closer, she found the tomb opened. Who could have ever arrived before her to pay respect to the precious body?

In front of the tomb, her gold grail of spices, dried fragrant flowers, and scented oil slipped through her shivering fingers and fell on the ground, pouring the perfumed ointment on the black soil. The heavenly scent spread. Adding hopelessness to her grief, she entered and realised that the tomb was empty. His body, the only trace remaining of him, was gone. It was a shock more traumatising to her than his death, a mysterious puzzle she could not solve.

Where was his body? Who had taken it? And why? She looked around for any clue, as her fear doubled by the second. Giving up on finding an explanation, but refusing to give in and leave, Marab sat down by the empty tomb, weeping. She did not know why she was still waiting, or what she was waiting for.

After some time, the heat of the sun, warming the awakening world, revived Marab's awareness. The breeze gently rummaged her curly locks under her shawl. Looking down, her tearless eyes beheld the blurry shadows of the trees. She heard people at a distance, working in the fields. She inhaled the perfume of her spilt ointment. She lifted her eyes and watched the birds diving into the clouds. Marab braced herself. The scene sparked her intuition. *If Yesham's words lived, would he ever die?*

Stubborn Hues

The sunlight came through the open window along with a gentle dewy breeze. It was not even six o'clock, but she could not go back to sleep. Her messy blonde hair framed her fatigued face on the pillow. She could not switch off her brain, so she decided to get up and make coffee. She blinked owlishly, as she struggled up, trying to find her way quietly through the enormous clutter in her bedroom. She went to the chaotic kitchen and turned on the coffee machine. She turned the TV volume down. He was still in bed, but whether he was sleeping or not, she was not sure. After last night, the last thing she wanted was to disturb him in any way.

Their relationship had been deteriorating recently, especially after a couple of serious disputes about the future of their life together. Lisa sat on the sloppy beige sofa. Tons of art magazines and newspapers were randomly thrown on the square coffee table in the tiny living room. In the corner stood her easel; dozens of scattered oil colour packs lay around it. Beside them, painted canvas frames were stacked against the canary wall.

She clutched her big coffee cup in her hand, while holding *La Repubblica* in the other and listening to the news at the same time. Yet she was only thinking about how to reconcile with him. Although the TV was not loud, it woke Roberto up. Despite all that had happened between them the previous evening, he still managed to sleep through the night. The second his eyes opened, he remembered everything. He got out of bed, showered, and got dressed. Lisa heard some movements coming from the room, wondering why it took Roberto so long to get ready that morning. He came out, willing a last attempt to talk to her again. He tried his best to be as gentle and fair as possible.

"*Buongiorno*," said Roberto. He prepared his lunch and put the lunch box in his briefcase, but he did not ask her what he should prepare for their dinner, as he usually did. He poured a cup of coffee for himself and walked into the living room. He sat down beside her on the sofa. She remained cold and aloof. He loomed closer and wrapped his muscular arm around Lisa's left shoulder, holding the cup with his right hand. His handsome face was freshly shaved, his thick brown hair glowed with gel, and his white shirt was perfectly ironed. He kissed her on the cheek, but she did not blink or turn her eyes away from the newspaper.

Roberto stayed silent and listened to the news. Lifting his arm away, he reclined back on the sofa. He asked, "How are you, darling?"

"Fine." She rubbed her forehead.

"I may have been a bit harsh last night, but that's because I care about you," he said.

"Of course." She threw the newspaper on the sofa and turned up the TV volume.

Roberto grabbed the remote and turned the TV off. "Listen! I'm saying it one last time. You need to fix your messy life and come down to Earth," he said.

"My messy life!" She shut her eyes.

"Honey, you're turning twenty-seven this summer, and you still don't have a decent job with a fixed monthly income." He slowly drank his coffee.

"I'm an artist. A painter. I'm preparing to open my own gallery. How many times do I have to tell you that?" Lisa punched the blue cushion.

"You have no idea what financial commitments you're facing. You don't know if it will be worthwhile, or if it will make any profit." He let out a harsh breath.

"Perhaps you can help me — if you really care — as you say." She rolled her eyes.

"I'm afraid you may actually lose money," he said.

"It's not about money for me." She looked away. "You'll never believe in my talent, will you? You always put me down and make me doubt myself." She slouched and hugged the cushion.

"You need to be realistic. Real life is something else. You need a job that pays good money. Your paintings won't pay your bills." He took the last sip of coffee and laid the cup on the table.

"Was I ever late in paying my share of the rent or any of our monthly expenses?" she asked, lips screwed angrily.

"You deserve a good profession, and you're able to get a good job with your degree. Plus, I'm tired of living in this mess. I hardly have room in this apartment for my own stuff. Your things are scattered in every corner of it. Look at all your junk all over the place!" Roberto raged.

"There we go. Be direct, say it straightforward. You don't want to live with me any longer."

"I love you, Lisa, and you know that," Roberto calmly said, "but this is not fair to me. I need my space, too. I have to leave now. I can't afford to be late for work."

Roberto rose from his seat. He put on his navy blazer and left, the powerful scent of his cologne permeating the room. Still sitting on the sofa, Lisa wondered what kind of job she could find with her Bachelor of Science degree in biology. She was not patient enough to be a teacher. She knew she was not the type of person who could be imprisoned in an office job, with strict working hours and a daily routine. Of all things in the world, this would be the most painful to her. Her freedom was valuable to her, and painting was the only thing in life that granted her this sense of liberty.

Lisa lay down, staring at the framed photo of them together on the corner table. They stood next to each other, he slightly shorter than she. She was still thinking about what he had just said. She could not determine where the problem was as long as she could support herself from her part-time job.

She worked at a famous restaurant in a tourist area by the Tiber River, where she made good money from tips; her salary was supplemented with her savings from the time when she had lived with her parents. She never asked herself how long her savings would last. Her only dream was to open her own gallery, and she was working hard to make it come true, but perhaps not hard enough.

She was about to burst into tears in an uncontrollable tantrum. To avoid falling apart, she needed to talk. She called three of her friends. None of them answered. "You think you have so many 'friends' but when you need them the most, they disappear," she muttered. Going through the contact list on her phone, she tried calling a few others, only to receive their voicemail.

Finally, she found no one to talk to except her mother. She called her. Teresa was very happy to hear from her daughter; it had been a month since Lisa had last contacted her. When she heard her troubled voice, Teresa asked her to come over for lunch before going to work in the evening.

Lisa got up and took a cool shower. Her short sandy blonde hair did not take a long time to dry on this hot day. She put on a colourful floral dress that had every shade in the rainbow on a Tuscan sun background. A bright gold chain surrounded her young neck, holding a pendant of the word, 'La Libertà'. An amber ring shone on her right hand. Round hoop gold earrings added femininity to her sharp-featured face. Her large hazel eyes with her skin, gorgeously tanned by the strong sun of Rome, painted the lovely portrait of a young lady full of youth and persistence. She put on her sunglasses and left to go visit her mother.

She walked the busy streets of Rome. Tourists were walking up and down the streets everywhere; there were hardly any inhabitants of Rome. It was noisy and crowded, but Lisa could not hear anything except her own voice talking in her head. It was quite a distance from her place to her mother's house, but she preferred walking to taking the bus. She needed to release some negative energy. Feeling the heat, she decided to stop on the way for a gelato to cool her down, releasing some of her anger with the lime gelato in a crispy cone.

The sweet and sour lime tasted like her relationship with Roberto. Despite sounding modern, at the end of the day, Roberto was a man. He needed a female helper, supporter, or perhaps follower. Lisa was far from being the right person to fill this role. Gradually, the gap between them became bigger every day; they talked less and spent even less time together. Still, their affection for each other remained.

Lisa was getting close to her parents' home, smelling her mother's famous home-baked pizza with tomato basil sauce and three kinds of cheese. The aroma filled the whole street. As she approached the door, she scented the fragrance of radiant roses and lilies, planted and maintained by her mother at the entrance. Teresa opened the door and held her tight; she truly missed her daughter.

The house was scrupulously clean. Everything was where it was supposed to be. The light blue carpet was freshly vacuumed, and the tiles were swept and mopped. The big statue of the Goddess Venus stood in the left corner of the living room, while an equal-sized statue of the Virgin Mary rose in the opposite corner, as they had since Lisa could remember. Above the sofa, a big tableau of the Mona Lisa was neatly centred on the grey wall. The antique wooden clock struck twelve and chimed. Stepping in toward the kitchen, Lisa could hear classical Italian songs, playing in the small cassette player beside the toaster on the kitchen counter. On the terrace, the sparrows chirped, flying between the hanging baskets of all colours of geraniums, begonias, and petunias.

They sat at the square mahogany table, where Teresa served her two slices of gourmet pizza, Caesar salad, and fresh orange juice. After all, what was more important for a mother than to generously feed her child? Whether to feed her food or love — both were necessary. Lisa managed to hide her pain and suppress her salty tears, but she could never fool her mother.

"How are your paintings coming along?" Teresa asked.

"I haven't painted for a while." Lisa sipped some orange juice.

"Why? You should actually start looking for a hall to rent for your gallery."

"We'll see." Lisa devoured another bite of pizza.

"Where did your enthusiasm go, Lisa?" Teresa asked, eyes crinkled.

"Apparently, what I paint is nothing extraordinary," said Lisa, rubbing the nape of her neck.

"Who told you that?" asked Teresa, glancing way. Lisa was busy chewing the pizza. "How is Roberto?" Teresa asked, forehead puckered.

"He's fine," Lisa said in an indifferent tone. "No, I am not sure," Lisa burst into bitter tears. "He doesn't want to live with me any more." Lisa covered her face with her hands.

"Oh dear, this must be heartbreaking." Teresa stood and held Lisa's head in her hand, while kissing it. "Do you know why? Did you talk?" concerned, Teresa asked.

"We've been doing nothing but talking. He can't put up with my messy life any more." Lisa wiped her tears and continued eating.

Roberto had a degree in economics and had managed to get a decent job as the Financial Advisor of the marketing department of one of the largest corporations in the fashion industry in Italy. His brain was as organised as his office at work. The only language he could understand was numbers and statistics. He needed to plan ahead, consider all probabilities, and prepare for every possibility. He had hoped for having a stable life in a neat house with Lisa but realised later that his dream might have been unrealistic.

"You're not pregnant, are you?" Teresa placed another slice of pizza in Lisa's plate.

"No, Mom, I'm not. Is that all you can think of? He got sick of living with me. He doesn't love me any more," Lisa groaned.

"I'm sorry, honey, but honestly, if he doesn't value your presence in his life, let him leave. He doesn't deserve you." Teresa crossed her arms and leaned back.

"No, Mom. I don't want him to leave. I love him," Lisa cried. She remembered it was noon — the time for Roberto's daily text message during his lunch break. She picked her phone from her purse, but there was no message from him. "I'm a loser. I'm not an artist. I'm nothing. Roberto is right." Lisa covered her eyes with a hand.

"I can't believe my ears, Lisa. I still have the artwork you made since you were in kindergarten. You were born to be a painter." Teresa's blue compassionate eyes glowed.

"You call those pieces of junk artwork!" Tears streamed down Lisa's cheeks. "No one believes in my art or my talent." She slammed her hand on the table.

"If you can't find anyone to believe in you, look in the mirror. Great artists became memorable for centuries not because their art was extraordinary, but because they believed their dreams and never gave up." Teresa stretched out her legs in front of her.

"He makes fun of what I paint. He calls my paintings 'trash of colours'." Lisa blubbered. She recalled Roberto's flattering compliments about her paintings when they had first met. How could a person change that much? She missed the Roberto with whom she had fallen in love two years earlier. The gentleman who had always made her feel valued.

"There's no right or wrong in art," Teresa said; "only what you think and how you feel matter."

"I'm not an artist, Mom." Lisa fiddled with her phone.

"Go to your room and look at the quote on the wall by Leonardo da Vinci — 'Simplicity is the ultimate sophistication'. You wrote it down yourself years ago."

"An artist is nothing without those who value her art." Lisa shook her head.

"Many famous artists lived all their lives unappreciated. Sometimes artists are ahead of their time," Teresa continued. "How many times did I tell you the stories of van Gogh, Bach, Kafka, Gauguin, and Edgar Allan Poe?" Teresa reminded her daughter of the bedtime stories she had told her when she was a child, while the latter was busy looking at Roberto's photos on her phone.

"I feel so worthless, Mom. I'm full of self-doubt. I don't want to lose Roberto," sighed Lisa, hands covering forehead.

"Whatever you do, don't stop painting. Start shopping around for a place. And if you need, find a second part-time job to make extra money. I'll help. I believe in you," Teresa promised.

Lisa slowly started to feel better, especially after the generous piece of rich tiramisu that her mother offered with a cup of tea after lunch. Despite her liberal thoughts, Teresa was a typical mother when it came to her family and home. She dedicated her complete time to making her home a comfortable place, raising her children and spending time with them.

Lisa helped her mother clean up after lunch. Finding herself thinking of Roberto, as if his scent was still in the air, she realised that she was confronted with a tough choice. Now she wanted to make it up to Roberto, but at the same time she needed to work harder on turning her dream into a reality. She checked her messages again, there was nothing from him.

It was nearly time for her to leave for her evening shift at La Luna restaurant. She hugged her mother and whispered in her ears, "Thank you, Mom. You're my inspiration."

"Every woman needs another woman to tell her how beautiful, intelligent, and strong she is. I'm happy to be that one in your life," Theresa said, holding her tight.

They said goodbye, and Lisa left. Her steps were more energetic and positive. She took the bus to the restaurant. She watched the tourists having fun in the sun, stunned by how amazing and full of history and beauty Rome was. As the bus approached the mighty Tiber, the sunrays' reflections in the water were breathtaking. The gentle breezes made the branches of the sycamore trees dance like ballerinas in an Italian opera house. "What a scene! I wish I could paint right now," she expressed.

She felt the urge to say "I love you" to Roberto right at that moment. She called him, but he did not answer. *What on earth is he doing?* She worried. Her concerns turned into vexation. *Now he is upset! As if he didn't hurt my feelings,* she raged.

She arrived at the restaurant and chatted with her colleagues. The restaurant was busier than usual that Friday night. Many customers were rich tourists from the States, and they were very generous with their tips. She worked her full shift until nine o'clock, but her supervisor asked her if she could work until midnight. Working extra hours meant more money. She could not say no. She texted Roberto that she would be late.

Lisa finished work. She left her high heels at the restaurant, as she did every day, and put on her comfortable runners. It was cool and breezy; she appreciated the quieter streets. She checked her messages, but there was no reply from Roberto. "What if something has happened to him?" Her fear grew. She had to do her best to reconcile with him. *We must reach a middle ground,* she thought. She arrived home, only to find it dark and empty. When she turned the light on, she found a note on the fridge with Roberto's handwriting, *Forgive me for quitting. I love you, but I need my freedom as much as you need your own. Roberto.*

Homeward

"Where am I? I want to go home. Let me go home, please," Lucy weakly voiced her wish, looking at the cold white ceiling of the hospital room with unblinking eyes. Barely able to see anything, she soon fell asleep again. Her breakfast tray was on the table, all the food untouched. Edmond sat silently by her bed, not feeling tired or bored. His arms were folded, and his eyes were shut.

The TV was on; he was not listening, but he always preferred the noise to the stabbing silence in the room. Since the ambulance took her to the hospital, all his days were similar, following the same routine. He woke up every morning at seven o'clock, took the bus to the hospital, stayed with Lucy all day until nine at night, and then took the bus back home.

Edmond noticed that Lucy's eyes opened again. "Can I get you anything?" he asked.

"I want to go home," she answered. By noon, Catherine arrived at Montreal General Hospital to give her father a break and spend some time with her mother, who barely felt the presence of anyone in the room. Edmond went downstairs to get a coffee.

Catherine stayed with Lucy. She turned the TV off and sat down, focusing on Lucy's chest slightly rising and falling. Catherine remembered many questions she still wanted to ask her mother, but she knew she would never get her answers. The nurse came in to check the morphine dose in the IV. "What a great man your father is," she said to Catherine. "Since your mother was admitted, he hasn't missed a single day."

"You think why he does that?" Catherine asked, fixing her eyes on Lucy.

"He loves her," the nurse concluded.

"He loves her," Catherine answered, "because she loved him first. You have no idea how devoted she was to him all the years of their marriage." Catherine went on and on, talking about her mother until the nurse had to stop her; she needed to help another patient in another room. As she left the room, the nurse whispered to her colleagues at the counter outside, "The dead get all the appreciation they missed when they were alive. Sad but true. We see this every day in this unit."

On his way back, Edmond met Cecile while she was hurrying to the elevator to come up to see her mother after she had finished a long work day. They came up to the hushed room, where Lucy was sleeping, and Catherine was gazing at her mother. The three of them sat down together and ate the sandwiches Cecile had brought with her. It was almost three o'clock in the afternoon; they were hungry.

Edmond appreciated the few minutes he could spend with his two daughters when they came to see Lucy. Their presence cheered him up immensely. He needed their affection to colour his grey days. Coming to the hospital had become a matter of habit for the three of them. Their shock and worry had gradually vanished from their minds, yet the feelings of helplessness and loss reigned over their hearts. There was nothing left that they could do for Lucy except be around her, as she peacefully lay there, reaching for the front gates of another realm.

It had started with a cold that she had suffered for a few days. It worsened and turned into a very bad flu for two days, until Lucy fell unconscious one day in the apartment.

After a few days of comprehensive medical tests and examinations, she was diagnosed with the most aggressive acute myeloid leukemia. For four months, she had received treatment in the hospital; her condition only deteriorated until her doctor decided to get her consent to stop the treatment. Everyone around her could see that the treatment was not helping, rather prolonging her suffering. She had just been moved to the palliative care unit the previous day.

After months of receiving the medication, Lucy's body became too frail to fight, her mind was ready to rest, and her soul was pleased to depart. Lying in the hospital bed, she was unconscious of the world of illusions, where her loved ones were still trapped. All her senses were sucked into a vacant site; she stood alone and could see or hear nothing but scenes, images, tones, and voices from her life since the very first day of it. She saw her joy and grief. She watched her successes, disappointments, wounds, and sins.

Contemplating the big picture, Lucy stopped trying to determine who was right, and who was wrong. She realised no one was right, and no one was wrong, but that people were all trying to do their best in the circumstances they had been given but had never chosen. She ceased blaming others or herself for everything that had gone wrong. Lucy attained the wisdom of not judging anyone, but rather justifying their actions, when she was left alone to be the only judge of her own deeds.

She was satisfied with the life she had lived, doing the best she could. She was content to leave with her loved ones the memories of her days among them and her influence on their lives. She knew she was not an angel or a saint. She was cognizant of her weaknesses and flaws, but she reached a point of self-purification that erased all bitterness. She was not resentful toward those who had hurt her; she forgave herself and them. Lucy succeeded in liberating herself from guilts and grudges. Life could only be understood backward. At last, everything made perfect sense to her. And all the problems and conflicts that had ruined her inner peace in the past, now seemed frivolously meaningless to her. With time, her wounds were cured. Her soul was comfortably at peace with the universe. Lucy passed the test.

"Guess what I brought with me!" Cecile said, a weary smile on her face. She opened her bag and took out a big envelope, "I've finally found them." They left Lucy alone in the room to sleep and went to the visitors' area to look at the pictures. Some pictures were of Lucy on her wedding day, with all the elegance of the late sixties. Many photos of the girls when they were babies until their graduation ceremonies brought laughter and memories from their childhood and adolescence.

Wishing Lucy was conscious to live this comforting moment, Edmond looked at the old photos of Lucy when she was young and beautiful until his phone rang. It was the human composting organisation, confirming the procedures. "I don't want to be buried in a coffin underground or cremated into ashes in a container. I want to become a tree," Lucy had willed the last time she could consciously speak.

Cecile originally was looking through the photos to find a good picture of their mother for the obituary, the funeral, and the eulogy cards that would be given away in memory of Lucy. They agreed on the best two photos of her: one in her youth, when she was twenty-four and one when she was a grandmother, two beautiful images at two different ages.

Catherine and Cecile left, and Edmond stayed by Lucy's side. Sometimes, he found himself talking to her, even though he knew she would not reply. Not only did he recall their sweet memories together, but also their hardships and disagreements, which normally did not last for a long time. Lucy was such a forgiving person, which made it harder for Edmond now to remember all the times he had disappointed her. She had simple requests that meant a great deal to her, like going with him to the movies or even for walks, but he was usually busy. Like a child, she was easy to hurt and easy to please. He regretted every word of love he could have said to her, but had not, and every caring gesture, which he had concealed. He wished she would wake up now and go home with him, so he could make it up to her.

He forgot about all the little things she had done that used to annoy him. What he had considered irritating in the past, now he saw as thoughtful and gracious. When she nagged him about going to the doctor, she cared for him. When she reminded him every second to fix something broken in the house, she needed his help. When she complained about some problems at her work, she wanted his support. When she asked to go out with him, she was keen on spending quality time with him. When she reproached him trying to explain why she was upset, she did not want to give up on their love. That was what he was only starting to realise.

Catherine and Cecile left the hospital, walked together to the metro station, agreed to start preparing for the funeral, and each went home. Cecile was going to prepare the stand and frame of Lucy's photos revealing her outer beauty, and Catherine was going to write the eulogy for her mother, describing her inner beauty and briefly telling her life story. Grateful, regretful tears were pouring from their eyes. They were both grateful that their mother had lived an honourable life and was ending it in a respectful way. Yet they were both regretful, but for different reasons.

On her way home, Cecile stopped by the photo studio and had the two photos professionally enlarged and printed. She bought two elegant wooden frames. Then, she went home and had dinner with her family. After cleaning up, she took the two pictures and frames and went to the living room. In the black-and-white picture, Lucy wore an elegant outfit and diamond earrings, her black hair up. Her kind brown eyes looked affectionately outward, and her smile motivated Cecile to seize whatever was left in her own life.

Looking at Lucy's pretty face, Cecile wondered whom she would run to when she would need two arms to hold her and two ears to listen. She pitied herself. Lucy was the only person who could comfort her when she was distressed, and made her feel loved and valued. Lucy knew how to remind Cecile of her positive traits and restore her composure. While her sister was a good friend, no one could take the place of Lucy in Cecile's heart. There were subjects she could hardly talk about with anyone but her mother.

Cecile had struggled with low self-esteem for years and talking to Lucy was her therapy. In silence, Sarah watched her mother for a while. "Mom, I'm going to see Granny tomorrow after my classes. I'll go straight from the university to the hospital," Sarah said, wringing her hands. "And Mom, you know I'm always here for you when you need to talk." Cecile and Sarah held each other tight in front of Lucy's framed photo.

Catherine walked home; she lived not too far away from the hospital. As the cool wind blew her long hair, Catherine heard echoes of her own voice yelling at Lucy. She blamed herself for having been cold and sometimes rude to her mother. She always believed Lucy was too naïve to give her advice. She rarely talked to her about anything, and when she did, Catherine often ended the conversation in anger, saying hurtful words to her mother. Catherine had lived all her life believing that she had the opposite personality of Lucy, and that they had very different opinions about everything.

Now, Catherine recalled situations when her mother had insightful wisdom very few people possessed. Her boyfriend had proven to be so irresponsible, disappeared suddenly and moved to Vancouver when she was preparing to move in with him. She had fought with her mother because of him, but in time Catherine learned that her mother was right. She remembered Lucy's comforting words of faith, trying to restore Catherine's hope when times were tough. Those words had meant little to Catherine in the past, but now they seemed priceless.

Catherine arrived in the quiet one-bedroom apartment. She made a sandwich and ate it with a glass of orange juice. Relieved to be able to sit down and rest her heavy body after a long day, Catherine turned on her laptop and started to write her mother's eulogy. 'Love Never Fails', was the title she chose, and "An angel went back to heaven," was her first sentence. She went on describing Lucy as a faithful daughter to her parents, a loving wife to her husband, an affectionate mother to her daughters and grandchildren, a loyal friend to her lifetime companions, and a dedicated teacher to thousands of students.

Catherine was so absorbed in writing that she hardly felt the strong kicking of her soon-to-be-born baby girl in her womb. She had decided to name her 'Faith' — the best word to summarise Lucy's life.

Edmond looked at his watch; it was nine o'clock. He turned the TV off, kissed Lucy's hand and forehead, put on his jacket, turned off the light, and took the elevator down. It was dark and cold. Feeling his wrinkled hands and bald head freezing, he realised that he had forgotten to take his gloves and hat out of the closet that morning. It was hard for him to believe that winter was already starting. It was Canada Day when the ambulance had taken Lucy to the hospital; he remembered seeing the red and white flags, fluttering in the wind all over the Vieux Port on the way to the hospital. It felt like time had stopped since then.

The bus took him around the streets of Montreal, passing by houses lit with big orange pumpkins and festooned black and white ghosts. Memories of Lucy and him preparing the small bags of goodies to give away to trick-or-treaters drew a baffled smile on his drained face. *It's very hard to comprehend the concept of someone whom you have known for so long not being there anymore,* he thought. Exhausted, he finally opened the door of the deserted apartment and sat down. As he sat looking at their forty-four-year-old wedding picture on the wall, he fell asleep in the armchair.

The Language of Love

In the early morning, she submitted her passport renewal application before going to work. Her new passport would be ready in four business days. She was not planning for any particular trip, but she was keen on renewing her passport. She felt comfortable knowing it was ready; she was looking for a reason to travel, preferably to somewhere she had never been before.

She took the underground metro to the British Council next to the wide old Nile. It was a warm and sunny winter day in Cairo as she entered the building and headed to the library. In late afternoon, a middle-aged gentleman approached her while she was leafing through some books. In a noticeable American accent he asked about specific books and DVDs in the art section on the history of drama in the Middle East, Egypt in particular. They talked for almost an hour. He provided as much information as possible, so she could help him find what he needed.

They also talked about many other irrelevant topics, one of which was the pendant attached to her necklace, which he admired greatly. She explained that it was the word *kemet* which meant 'Egypt' in the Ancient Egyptian language, written in Hieroglyphic alphabet. She elaborated on the topic and concluded, "Coptic was the last phase of the ancient Egyptian language, written in Greek alphabet. The same evolved spoken ancient Egyptian language was spoken by all Egyptians until the twelfth century." She stood straight, holding a book with her arms against her chest.

His eyes widened, as he shifted from one foot to another, astonished by the knowledge she provided for that simple comment on her necklace. "WOW! I am impressed," he said. His pupils dilated.

"I am a linguist," she quipped. They both chuckled. At last, she had all the information written down, as well as his email address. She promised she would do her best to find what he needed and that he could collect the titles the following day. She gave him her business card: Hirini Soliman, Library Manager. "Thank you, Ms. Soliman," he said, looking down at the business card.

"Hirini. Please call me Hirini," she grinned. She could not help telling him that *hirini* meant 'peace' in Coptic, and that it was her mother's choice to name her Hirini.

"A beautiful name and a beautiful meaning," he added, his eyes glittering with admiration. As he was leaving he explained that her library was a last resort after he had looked in many libraries and bookstores in Cairo. He thanked her sincerely and left.

Joseph Merkin was the most mysterious American Hirini had ever met. There was something divergent about him. He sounded undoubtedly American, but he was somewhat different. She could hardly guess his origin. His white skin and straight black hair suggested that he might have been of Italian or Spanish descent, yet his last name did not. His brown eyes were wide, with thick eyelashes, and reflected the smile on his lips. He was exactly her height, even though she was not a tall woman. She thought he could be her age or younger.

Hirini spent the rest of the day looking in archives, trying to locate everything that could possibly be related to the topic he was researching. She worked late after hours preparing the titles for him, reading many of the sections.

It was important for her to find a good reason to contact Joseph the following day. On her way home, she stopped at *Balady* to buy a falafel sandwich for dinner. Exhausted, she arrived at her spacious apartment in central Cairo, where she had grown up and still lived until that day. She went straight to her bedroom.

"In the Beginning Was the Word," was written in artistically calligraphic letters, surrounded by randomly scattered alphabets of every writing system known to humans. The richly crafted wood plank hung on the beige wall in front of the bed. Above it was an enormous colourful papyrus portrait of Queen Nefertiti, set in an antique bronze frame. Hirini pulled the elegant rose duvet aside and plunged into her bed, thinking of enigmatic Joseph.

It occurred to her that it was time to read her last letter. She rose and opened her closet. She picked the brown leather briefcase, where she kept every significant piece of paper she owned. She squatted on the floor, looking for it. A nostalgic smile brightened her face when she found her old notebook that she had kept since her college days. "A linguist is a person who realises, through studying the origins of languages, that all people are one," she had written on the first page.

On one of the pages was the family tree of the languages of the world, starting on top with Indo-European, Afro-Asiatic, and Sino-Tibetan. She could not help reading every single line on the chart, observing how they all traced back to one single origin. But this was not the notebook she was looking for.

She checked everything in there until she saw the photos envelope. She sighed and grinned; she knew what was there — a world of memories. *Relationships!* She mumbled. She tried to ignore it, but her stubborn hand opened it and picked one picture at a time, starting with the oldest.

The first photo was of Emad and her at the University of Cairo. She had thought that he was the love of her life, not realising he was only the first. The second picture was of Richard, the British lawyer who worked in Cairo. He was fond of her lively positive nature, and she was attracted by his maturity and sophistication — and of course, his British accent. The third photo she picked was with Olivier, her young French teacher at the French Cultural Centre in Cairo. She laughed; she remembered how funny he was.

Hirini put the envelope back and searched until she found the notebook. She opened it, flipping the pages to where she had written letters to her future self at different stages of her life. She read the last one, which she had written three years earlier after her parents had passed away within a few months from each other.

The letter reassured Hirini and reminded her that in many past situations things had usually worked together for good, one way or another. She missed her parents. She had been alone for quite some time now. She rose and put the briefcase back on the shelf. It was 9:00 PM. She went and took a warm bath, listening to some old Egyptian songs. She then prepared her clothes for the next day and went to bed, looking forward to seeing Joseph.

When Hirini arrived at work the next day, she went straight to her office rather than chatting with her colleagues, as she did every morning. Turning on her computer, she opened the list of titles. She wrote an email, letting him know what she had found.

When she finished the last line of her email and before hitting the send button, her office phone rang. "Good morning. Hirini speaking," she answered.

"Good morning, Hirini. This is Joseph. Sorry, I'm calling so early."

"Hi Joseph. No problem at all. How are you?" she said, in a relaxed tone. "I was writing an email to you. It has a list of all the books and DVDs I've found for you. You may stop by and pick them up, whenever you can."

In the early afternoon, Joseph knocked gently on her office door and allowed himself to come in and sit down on the chair in front of her desk. They talked for another hour. He thanked her for the books and said that he would spend the evening checking them, and return them when finished. Before leaving, he asked if she was interested in going out for a drink after work. Without giving it a second thought, she said, "I'd love to."

Hirini was elated as she prepared to meet Joseph. She put on her crimson sweater, her knee-length A-line jean skirt, a sage scarf, and flat shoes. She wore simple, natural makeup, and alluring herbal perfume. Her image in the mirror resonated with the statue of the Goddess Isis on the dresser.

She arrived on time at the Left Bank Café, where they were to meet at 7:00 PM. Dressed in a dark green shirt and jeans, he sat at a small table beside a corner window overlooking the Nile. He asked her how the rest of her day had been, and she entertained him with stories until the waiter interrupted to ask what they wanted to drink. She asked for a tomato juice, and looking at the waiter he asked for a banana milkshake in an almost fluent Palestinian dialect.

Surprised, Hirini exclaimed, "You speak Arabic!"

"Palestinian," he said.

"I thought you were American. Where did you learn Palestinian?" she asked.

"I was born and raised in Alabama until I was ten, then I moved with my parents to Jerusalem, where I learned Palestinian as part of my daily life."

"Are your parents Palestinian?" Hirini asked, eyebrows raised.

"No, they're American," he answered.

Suddenly, his mobile phone rang. He looked at it and apologised sincerely to Hirini. He had to take this long-distance call; it was his sister from Jerusalem. He started his phone conversation in a language completely unknown to Hirini. Curious, she listened attentively to guess what language it was, but she could not really tell. When he finished, she asked, "What was this language?"

"Hebrew," he answered.

That was a mind-blowing shock to Hirini. *A linguist who spent four years at the university studying the bloody language family tree could not identify the language of a next-door country! What a shame!* She rebuked herself. To that extent, the media had succeeded in deleting the existence of the State of Israel not only from the map, but also from people's brains.

Israel did not exist in Egyptian media, drama, or school curricula for students to learn, except as the hated enemy. Until that day, the Middle East map in the social studies books called this tiny piece of land 'Palestine'. Israel's name was only heard in the news, reporting the horrible crimes the Israeli government committed against helpless Palestinians. The government claimed to have made the peace treaty with Israel in the seventies after the Egypt-Israeli war, but the reality was, the culture and mentality of people in Egypt and the Middle East refused its existence.

All these reflections sparked in Hirini's head for a few seconds. Trying to collect her thoughts and hide her confusion, she resumed, "How on earth did I miss that? You grew up in Jerusalem; of course, it's Hebrew." Her back shrunk, as she smoothed down her skirt.

"My parents are Jewish American," he said.

"Oh yes, it all makes perfect sense now," she stuttered, heart pounding. "I am very embarrassed that I couldn't recognise Hebrew. Can't believe I missed that," she panted, looking down at her sweaty hands. She twisted her turquoise silver ring.

"They decided to move to Israel for good twenty-five years ago."

Very quickly, she did the math in her head, realising that he was one year younger than her. The tomato juice and the banana milkshake were served. Hirini's hands hugged the cold glass, trying to cool off. She cleared her throat and continued, "So, your mother tongue is American, while Hebrew is considered your native language. As for me, Arabic is my mother tongue, while Coptic is my native language; it's the language of my heritage and real identity."

"Well, yeah, you could say both English and Hebrew are equally my mother tongue."

"What you speak is American, not English," she said.

"I thought they were the same thing." He sipped some of his drink.

"American is a dialect of its own," Hirini explained. "You even spell words differently in the States." She winked.

"If you say so. I'm not going to argue with a linguist." His gaze dipped to her neck.

"You better not," she grinned, "Do you know how to read and write Arabic?" she asked.

"I do read and write Arabic," he answered.

"How did you learn it? At school?" She grew inquisitive.

"No, not at school. I had private lessons at first. Then, I continued teaching myself by reading Arabic newspapers and listening to the Arabic radio."

"Although language was originally meant to be a means of communication to connect people, it ended up being a barrier between them," Hirini contemplated. "Yet I believe that a native language to a people is their true heritage, and if they lose it, they lose with it their identity, history, independence, and sense of belonging."

"That's exactly what Hebrew means to the Jews," Joseph agreed.

"I wish the Egyptians had looked at it the same way and not let their language and identity die," she said.

Hirini and Joseph shared a passion for languages, but in two different ways. Detail-oriented, Joseph was interested in the definite aspects of a language like vocabulary, slang, accents, and dialects. Hirini, however, was more absorbed in the bigger picture rather than the details. The origins of languages and the linguistic evolutions in different cultures were the most interesting topics for her to learn about.

She continued, "You know, Hebrew and Aramaic, the original Palestinian language, come from the same language family: The Afro-Asiatic, and so do Arabic and Coptic."

"Interesting! I always thought Coptic was different," he said.

"Hebrew, Aramaic, and Arabic are sister languages, but Coptic is their cousin," she explained. "It is like, for example, English, French, and Spanish. They all belong to the Indo-European family, but French and Spanish are sisters, coming from the Italic family, while English is their cousin, descending from the Germanic family."

"I see." He stared at her unrelentingly. "Do you speak Coptic then?" Joseph asked, stirring his milkshake with the straw.

"The only way I could speak Coptic would be if I talked to myself." She bowed her head. "No one speaks Coptic any more, sadly. But I do read and write Coptic." She took a sip from her juice.

"Oh yes, you explained how the Coptic language gradually disappeared, but so did Hebrew. Hebrew was revived in the twentieth century after almost seventeen centuries of not having been spoken."

"I know. That was a miracle," said Hirini, hands clasping the glass of juice.

"All these years, the Hebrew language was preserved through prayer books in synagogues all over the world, but nobody actually spoke it."

"Same as Coptic. It has been preserved only in the Egyptian churches as the language of hymns and prayers. But the truth is many words in the spoken Egyptian dialect are originally Coptic."

"Did you learn Coptic at school?" Joseph rested his chin on his palm.

"No. Ironically, Coptic is not taught at Egyptian schools." She gave a wry smile.

"You must have learned it at church, then," assumed Joseph, head tilted.

"No. I learned Coptic at home. My mother was a professor of Egyptology."

Hirini's discomfort slowly vanished, and she gradually opened up to Joseph. Her unease and nervousness were overpowered by their amusing conversation. *Maybe the Israelis are not that scary after all!* She thought. Joseph did have many Palestinian friends in Jerusalem, so talking to a Middle-Eastern was not a reason for him to feel any anxiety. Plus, he evidently had a soft spot for Egypt.

"Are you Coptic?" he asked. "If you don't mind me asking."

"Well, it depends what you mean by 'Coptic'," Hirini punned.

"As far as I understand, it means Christian Egyptian. Doesn't it?"

"This is an incorrect connotation that gradually became widely accepted or rather enforced for political reasons. But the real meaning of the word 'Coptic' in the Egyptian language has nothing to do with beliefs or religions. Coptic is a language. A nationality. It simply means 'Egyptian'." Hirini fiddled with her dangling coral silver earring.

"Alright then, are you a Muslim Coptic or a Christian Coptic?" Joseph persisted.

"What difference does it make?" Hirini answered with a question.

"It doesn't make any difference. I am just curious," he replied.

"Well, stay curious, then," she teased him. "You'll figure it out on your own." She winked.

"You're not veiled. So maybe you're not a Muslim," he guessed.

"*Hijab* has nothing to do with religion, by the way," said Hirini, arms crossed. "It's all politics; it's just a way to discriminate against the non-Muslim women and supress the Muslim ones, brainwashing them into believing they choose it freely. Maybe religion is politics after all." Hirini tapped her fingers on the table.

"You're not wearing an Islamic pendant, nor a cross either, like most Egyptian women." He stared at her necklace.

"I assume by now you can already tell that I'm different from many women, let alone the Egyptian ones." Her flirtatious laughter clinked, and so did her silver ring, striking the tall glass between her hands.

Hirini's persistence in bewildering Joseph and her naughty stubbornness captivated him, while his noticeable rare talent in mastering different languages mysteriously attracted Ms. Linguist. She was impressed by his linguistic skills, and he was intrigued by her immense knowledge of the history of languages and cultures. They both loved each other's sense of humour and enjoyed shared laughter. He listened to the rich information coming out of Hirini's beautiful lips. He grew so curious that he had an irresistible desire to collect her puzzle pieces and discover everything she was trying to hide.

Joseph excused himself to go to the washroom. When Hirini had some time alone to reflect, she realised the dilemma she was in. *A Jew! What have I done to myself?* she feared. She had never known Jewish people in her life. By her generation, all Jewish Egyptians had left Egypt for Israel, Europe, or North America. There were almost none of them left. As much as she loved his personality, she felt the complication this experience might bring her.

With her chin resting on her palm, she watched him coming back to the table. Looking at his smiling eyes, she forgot the tension his ethnicity could cause and found herself opening up to him again. Joseph sat down and said, "I'd like to thank you again for your help in finding the titles for me."

"My pleasure. Tell me, what do you need them for?" she asked.

"I am a journalist. I need them for a series of articles I write about the image of Jews in Egyptian drama."

"This is an interesting topic." She gasped, feeling the unease anew.

"Great. Hirini, I'm gonna tell you what I've been thinking about. In short, I am also a professional photographer, and I was wondering if you would accept to be my model for some photos in historical places in Egypt."

"A model? Me?" Hirini said, narrow-eyed.

"Yes. I'm opening my gallery in Tel Aviv in two months, and I'm planning to have a section on Egypt. That's another reason why I'm here. I need a volunteer to be my model, and she has to be Egyptian. And by the way, I want to tell you that you are uniquely beautiful."

Hirini's name, face, and body were evocations of her identity. Her face was sharp, thin, and well-formed, featuring a dark complexion, big dark brown eyes, nicely shaped black eyebrows, curled black eyelashes, long nose, a wide mouth with luscious lips, hiding two lines of pearl teeth behind them, and long curly black hair. Her body was appropriately proportioned, her soft curves a lovely silhouette of the female body. "I need some time to think about it," Hirini said. She bit her lip and glanced away.

"I'm leaving in four days. You have to give me an answer tomorrow morning."

Joseph hoped her answer would be 'yes'. To Hirini, however, it felt like a very difficult decision. She only had a few hours to decide. Her heart was jumping for joy, thinking of the fun she could have for four days in his company. Still, her mind was swinging between yes and no, feeling worried and concerned.

It was getting late, and they had to leave, although they did not want to. To Joseph's surprise, Hirini paid for her own drink, but he did not really mind. "It's not a big deal. I could've paid it," he said.

"When ladies let men pay for them, they give society a good reason to justify that it's normal for men to earn more money than women," she respectfully argued.

They left and walked by the prehistoric Nile until they reached her apartment building. Nothing could infatuate her more than going for a walk by the water at night. Egyptian songs, from the *feluccas* sailing the Nile, warmed up the cold night. The lights of the busy Cafes and restaurants by the river brightened the dark skies. Couples and groups of friends walked down the streets. Yet all the noise of Cairo could not distract Hirini and Joseph from concentrating on each other's breaths and glances. They stood in front of her apartment building and talked again for thirty minutes. It was chilly, but they were both warm.

Saying good night, Joseph walked to the underground station. He was impressed by Hirini's personality. He was confident enough not to let himself be intimidated by how independent she was. The fact that she was independent not only financially, but socially and emotionally as well, was top on the list of traits he liked about her.

Hirini went up and entered her apartment. She still could not get over her disappointment that she had not recognised the sound of Hebrew. Everything that happened that evening made her think about something she had never been interested in before — the Arab-Israeli conflict in the Middle East. She started to question why there was a conflict in the first place.

How could the Muslim Arabs deny the Israeli's right in the land, while they had in their Quran accounts of the Israelis inhabiting that land tens of centuries earlier? Similarly, the Jewish Torah mentioned the people of Palestine and that they lived in the same area. Until when would the Israelis and the Palestinians continue to live in war and let people from both sides be killed and children be orphaned? Until when would they let fear and hatred triumph?

Lost in thought, she heard the phone ringing. It was Sally letting her know that she and two other friends were planning to go to the movies the following evening and asking if Hirini would like to join them. "I'd love to come, but I'll tell you for sure tomorrow morning," Hirini said to her. They talked for thirty minutes without her mentioning one single word about Joseph. After all, she did not need to hear any comments to inflame her fears. She knew how most Egyptians would think about an awkward relationship like hers with him.

Tired, she ran a warm bath, thinking about no one but Joseph and how different he was. Afterwards she collapsed into bed. Unable to fall asleep, she rose, and opening her computer searched for information about Israel and Palestine.

She found Israeli websites with hateful articles against the Palestinians by fanatic Jews. She remembered the hate speech against the Jews that she had heard all her life from the microphones of the mosques in Cairo. *The hatred is mutual then,* she concluded. Just when she started to lose hope in finding something to comfort her, she found archaeological and genetics research papers about the two nations.

She read for about two hours. Her own conclusion was that both cultures shared similar origins and had lived in this area for thousands of years. Their cultures were intermingled. Although a large number of Israelis had emigrated and lived in other countries all over the world for centuries, a fair number of them had stayed and never left.

She wondered why the Israelis and Palestinians could not live side by side in peace, each in their own state. *How could they ever ignore the fact that Hebrew and Aramaic were sister languages emerging in the same geographical area?* she wondered. She suddenly laughed, when she learned that the year marked the silver jubilee of the Egypt-Israel Peace Treaty signed in the late seventies. Feeling a little more comforted, she went back to bed. She fell asleep, <u>Goddess of The Nile</u> lying on the night table beside her bed.

The next day, she called Joseph in the morning and accepted to be his model. Hirini decided to listen to her heart and let it convince her mind that everything was going to be alright. Together, they spent the most adventurous three days, one day in the Roman and Greek monuments in Alexandria, another day in the historical Christian and Islamic sites in old Cairo and the pyramids of Giza, and the last day in the pharaonic temples in Luxor.

Joseph took breath-taking photos of her beauty and Egypt's history. The more she talked to Joseph and spent time with him, the more she felt comfortable and relaxed.

They grew more intimate by the minute. They realised other common interests they shared. More importantly, they also discovered their differences. In spite of having similar personality traits, they still had different opinions and political positions, yet they both could understand the opposite point of view and know where it came from. They respected their differences while cherishing their similarities.

At last, the three days were over, and it was time for him to leave for Israel. She insisted on seeing him off at the airport. When it was boarding time for his flight, Joseph managed to find a hidden corner where no one was around and gave Hirini a hug to say goodbye. He buried his hands in her hair and stole one last quick kiss from her succulent lips. She let herself melt in his affectionate arms. His last words were, "In two months will be the inauguration of my gallery in Tel Aviv, where all your pretty photos will be exhibited." On her way back, she picked up her new passport, already planning her next trip.

About the Author

Reader of people and books
Writer of stories and poems
Painter with words and colours
Listener to souls and songs.

Lina Girgis believes in changing lives through art. Egyptian by birth, Canadian by choice, Lina has lived her life on two continents, which is reflected in the multiculturalism of her stories.

Holding a Bachelor of Arts degree in English, Lina treasures English literature and culture. She completed a Professional Writing Certificate specialising in marketing and public relations to supplement her passion for writing.

She has been writing short stories in English since 2014. The first story in <u>Liberation</u>, A Glimpse Inward, was published in the online literary magazine *The Write Launch* in March 2019. Lina also writes poems in Egyptian, some of which have been published in the biweekly Egyptian-Canadian newspaper, *Al-Ahram Elgdeed*.

Happy and honoured to be a woman, Lina finds spiritual inspiration through nature. As the mother of two amazing young people, she respects the visions of the new generation.

In her writing Lina strives to illustrate women's feelings, define their thoughts, and express their views with insight and honesty.

CPSIA information can be obtained
at www.ICGtesting.com
Printed in the USA
BVHW071542190920
589122BV00003B/8

9 781989 048603